healthy meals

L♥VE TO COOK

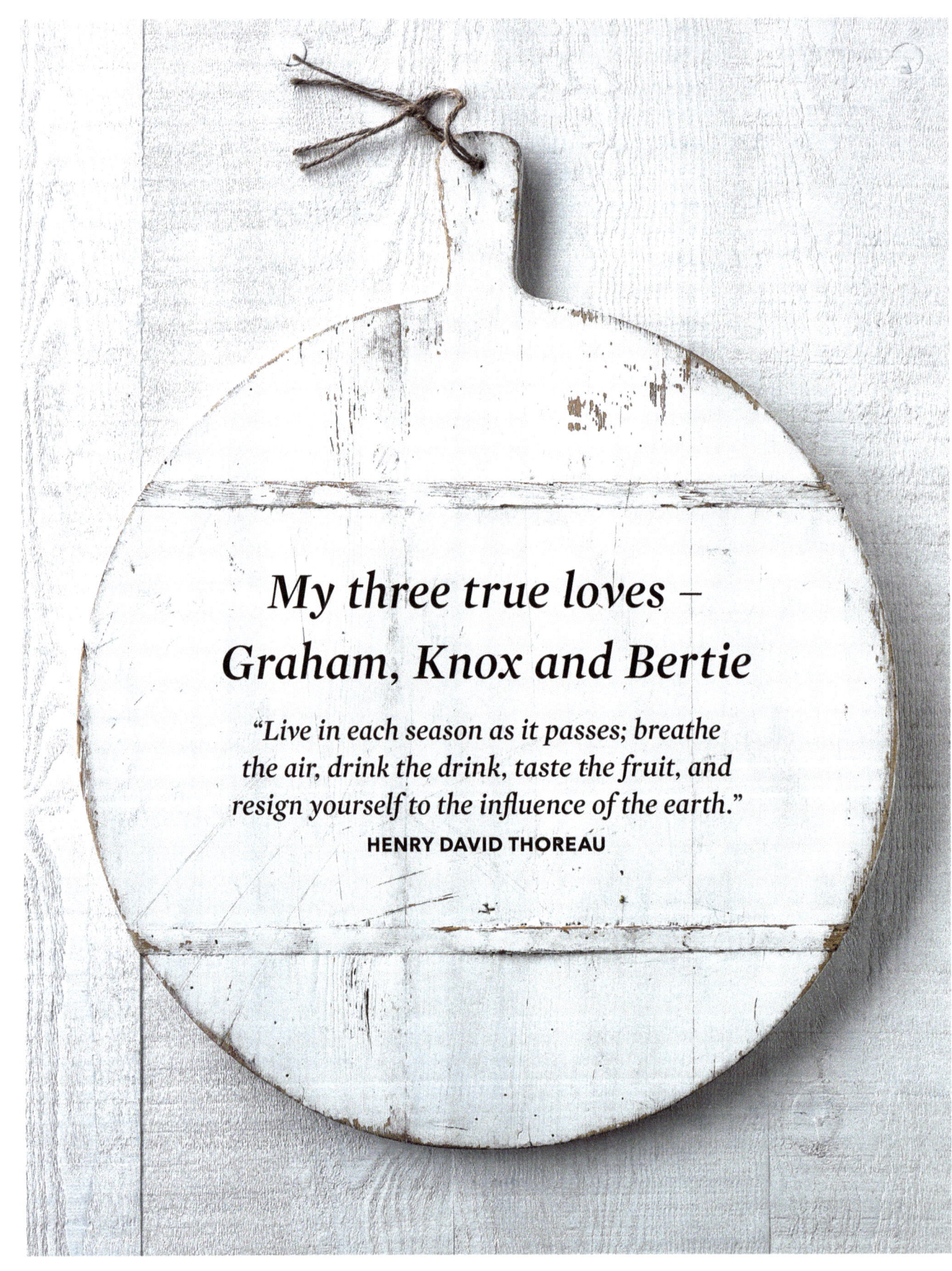

My three true loves – Graham, Knox and Bertie

"Live in each season as it passes; breathe the air, drink the drink, taste the fruit, and resign yourself to the influence of the earth."

HENRY DAVID THOREAU

love to cook

HEALTHY MEALS

Tracey Pattison

contents

HEALTHY MEALS

Introduction / **7**
Learning to Love To Cook / **8**
Uncomfortable in the Kitchen? / **10**
A Healthy Meal / **12**
Children Loving Vegetables / **14**
About My Recipes / **17**
Tomato Sauce / **21**
Stewp / **35**
Roasting Chicken / **49**
Slow-cooking Lamb / **63**
Stir-frying Chicken / **77**
Char-grilling Steak / **91**
Salad Sides / **105**
Smash Sides / **121**
Vege Sides / **137**
Index / **152**
About Tracey / **154**

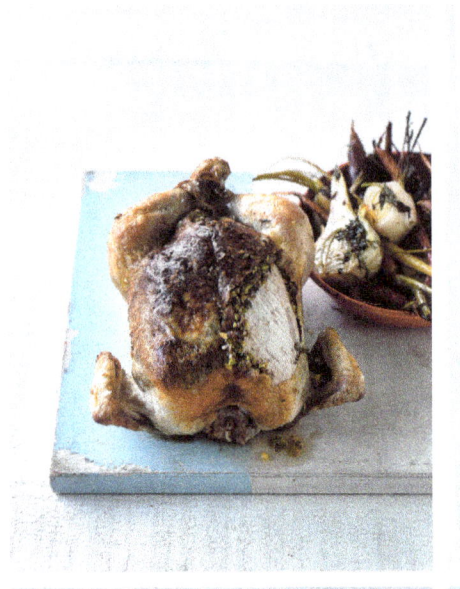
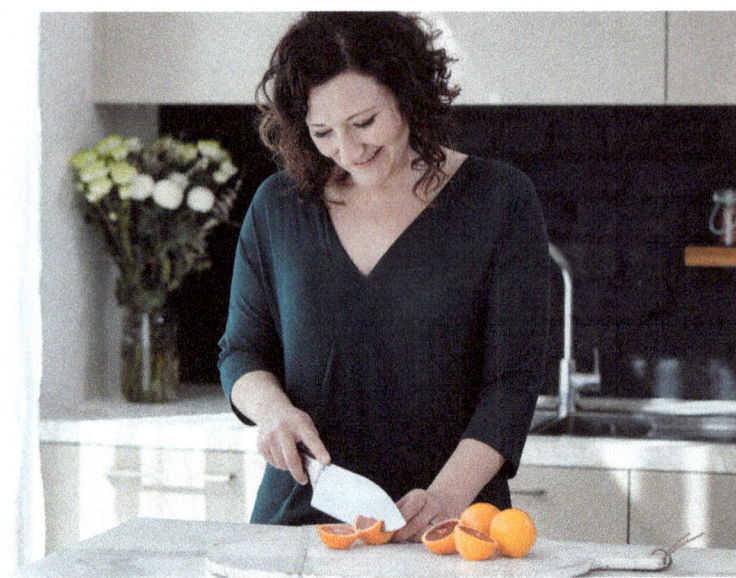
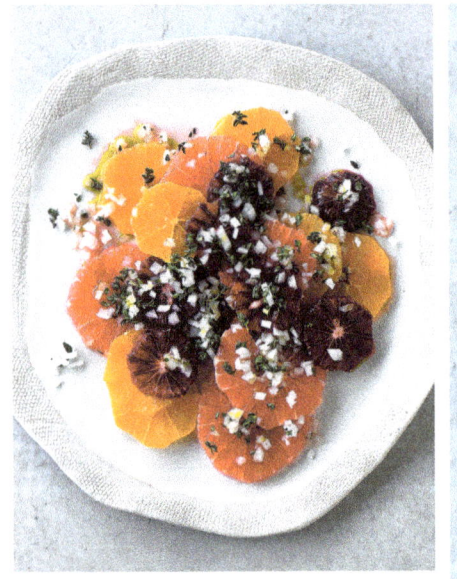
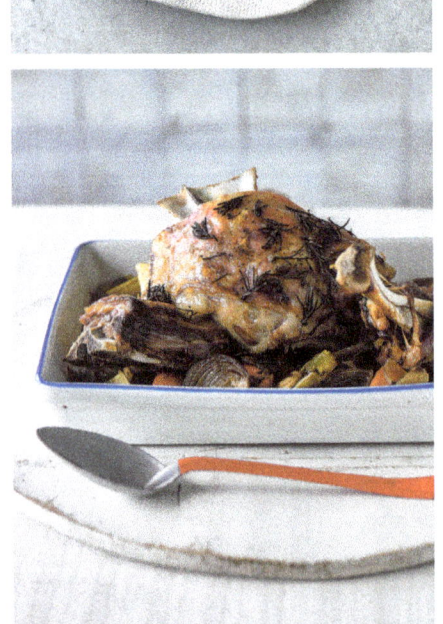

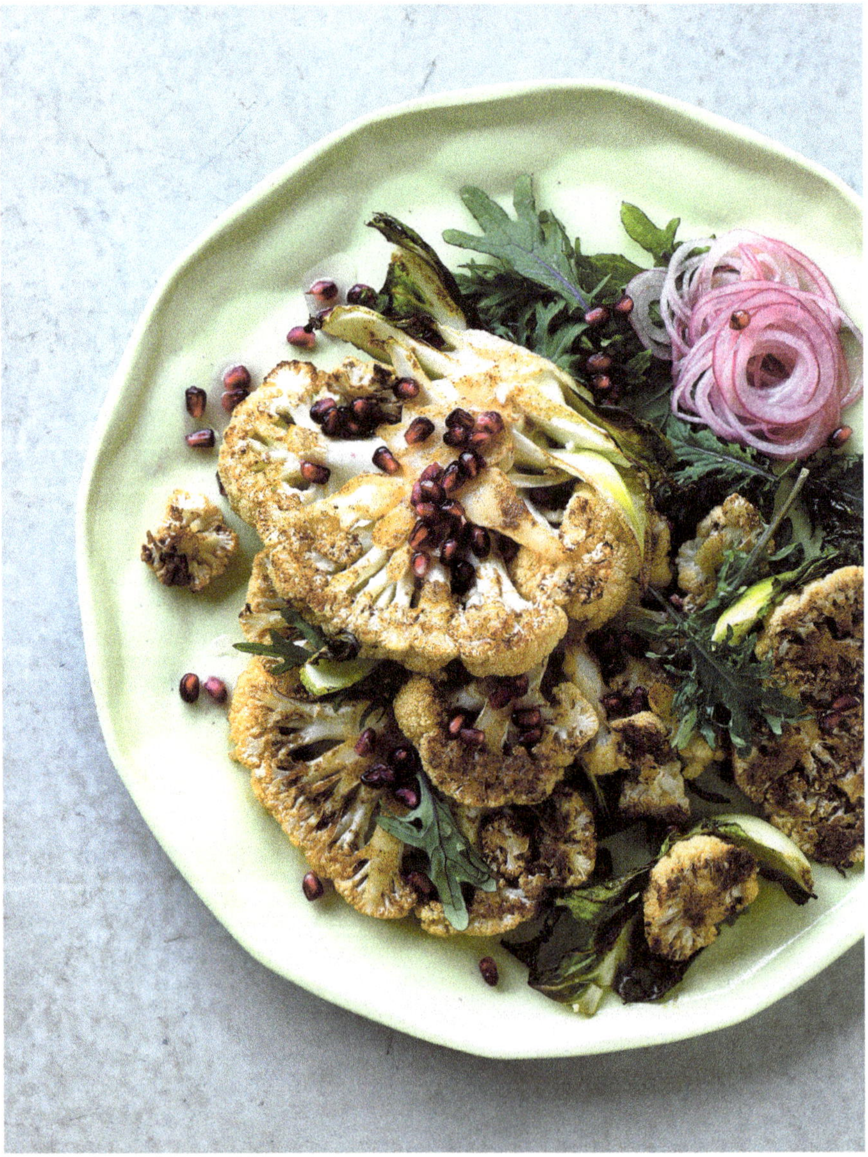

Introduction

Do you find cooking a chore or are you stuck in a food rut? Does the kitchen make you feel uncomfortable or are you looking to save money, improve your health and get your children eating at mealtimes?

My cookbook can help you. The recipes in this book are made with love on a daily basis directly from my own kitchen. It's packed with tried and tested, great tasting, healthy recipes which are grounded by my two decades of professional food publishing experience.

As a mother of two young children I understand how difficult mealtimes can be so I am giving you my top 6 basic healthy recipes and provided variations on each of them, giving you an abundance of meals to choose from that are specifically designed for families, people needing inspiration and those looking to better their health. Meaning that there is something in here for everyone.

There are over *530 handy cooking tips, delicious recipes, side dishes and pieces of practical cookery advice* to empower you in the kitchen.

My intention for this cookbook is to provide inspiration and guidance at each turn of the page, giving you the confidence in the kitchen you deserve, so that you can truly learn to Love To Cook *Healthy Meals* and in turn live a holistic, healthy life.

With L♥VE,

Tracy ♡

Tracey Pattison

LEARNING TO LOVE TO COOK

As a qualified Health Coach (IIN) my holistic approach to food means that I believe the foundation to great health begins with learning to Love To Cook. Getting back to the basics in mind, body and kitchen.

Lets get honest here, why don't you love cooking?

IS IT A CHORE?

If you find that everyday you loathe the idea of having to cook and find it is just one extra item on your long to-do list, then here are three simple time-saving suggestions to make the process of preparing home cooked meals just that much more enjoyable:

♥ **Get organised**

Yes, this may seem a lot of work initially but trust me. Spend the time on a weekend afternoon to plan your meals up to a month ahead – work out what recipes you will cook over the month and then write them into your diary or on an easily visible calender.

♥ **Shop wisely**

Once you have chosen your recipes for the month, write up your shopping lists. Do one big dry store shop at the start of the month, then do a weekly fresh food shop according to how you have planned your recipes over the month. Not only will you save a lot of time by not having to 'duck into' the shops for last minute food items but you will save money too by sticking to a shopping list.

♥ Batch cook

Another big time saver is batch cooking. Pick out some of your favourite freezer-friendly recipes chosen for the month and double or triple them, then portion, label and freeze. All you have to do is re-heat your chosen meal at the end of a very busy day.

IN A FOOD RUT?

We all get caught up in our busy lives from time to time and find that there can be weeks where you have cooked the same meals week-in-week-out. Did you make Bolognese 3 times last week? Here are three simple ways you can get inspired again and break boredom in the kitchen:

♥ Cookbooks

Sometimes all it takes is a lovely pictured meal from a gorgeous cookbook to inspire you. Use cookbooks as tools to stretch your imagination about how you can prepare your favourite meat, chicken, fish or vegetarian meal.

♥ Visit a farmers market

Walking around a Farmers Market will always create inspiration. Being surrounded by all the gorgeous colours and smells of fresh produce and then getting the chance to talk directly to the people who have produced, reared or grown what you are about to purchase will have your head buzzing with excitement to get back into the kitchen with your new purchases.

♥ Talk food

Surround yourself with people who genuinely love to cook and by default you will strike conversations around food. Ask for their favourite go-to meals, swap success recipes, laugh about failures and see what inspires others to cook.

UNCOMFORTABLE IN THE KITCHEN?

Perhaps holding a knife doesn't feel comfortable to you or maybe you just can't ever seem to cook rice without it becoming gluggy. The fear of stepping foot in the kitchen is valid as it is hard to invest time, money and energy into a task that may fail. Here are three basic ways you can help expand your comfort level when stepping into the kitchen:

- ♥ **Take time.** Spend some time to master a basic skill or particular recipe. Go on-line to my site *www.getfoodfit.com* for lots of handy hints and tips for cooking success in the kitchen. Watch short video tutorials and practice, practice, practice. All you need is the time and space to allow yourself to learn and succeed.

- ♥ **Bring love.** Set your kitchen up so that you want to be in there cooking. Have your favourite music playing, light some candles, have pots of fresh herbs on the windowsill or a vase of your favourite flowers. Make it an inviting space so that you are naturally drawn in and it becomes a sanctuary for you.

- ♥ **Set yourself up.** Organise your kitchen in a way that supports how you like to cook. Perhaps you find it easier to have your pans hanging from the wall or maybe a large glass jar filled with all of your favourite wooden spoons helps you feel at ease. Organise your cupboards and draws and cluster like items together such as bowls, measuring cups and spoons. By taking the time to set yourself up in the kitchen means that you can easily find what you need when you need it, making the process of cooking just that much more enjoyable.

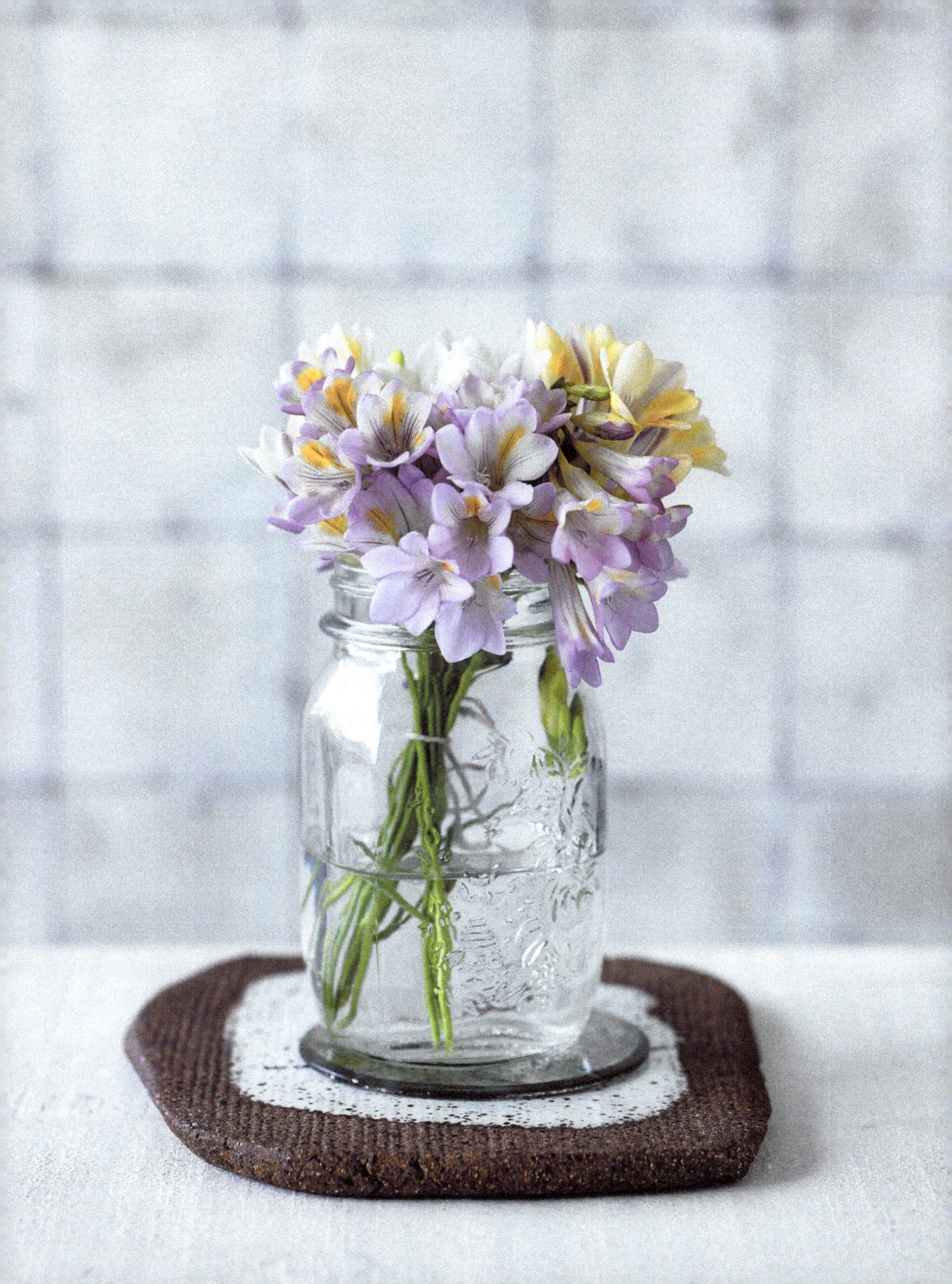

A HEALTHY MEAL

A healthy meal is more than just cooking and cooking is more than just preparing food and applying heat. It is about providing nourishment for yourself and those around you so that you can sustain the energy needed to get through the busyness of day-to-day living, support your body so that you can ward off illness and more importantly provide a loving act of self-care as a reward for what you achieve through the day.

My holistic cooking and eating rituals practiced daily:

- Be truly **thankful** for the food you are able to purchase and are able to eat.

- Practice **gratitude** towards the farmers, the earth, the environment and those who have produced, reared or grown the food available to you.

- Purchase **fresh** fruits and vegetables when in season. In-season produce tastes better, is more nutritionally sound and cheaper to purchase.

- Eat the **rainbow**! Select a rainbow of colour when purchasing and cooking your fruits and vegetables, choose something from each category of green, purple/blue, red, yellow/orange, and brown/white. By doing this, you are getting varied nutrients and also making your dishes more appealing to the eye.

- ♥ Try to purchase **locally grown** produce, ethically raised poultry and meats from your nearest farmers market.

- ♥ If your budget can support it purchase **organic** or bio-dynamic produce, poultry and meats. If you can only afford a very small amount, a great place to start is with organic eggs. Then simply add small amounts of poultry and meats. You can also extend your poultry and meat meals out by adding dried pulses and beans – you then get the best of both worlds!

- ♥ Always purchase **sustainable seafood** to ensure what goes on your plate has had minimal impact on fish populations, marine wildlife and ecosystems.

- ♥ Get those you **love** beside you and involved in the cooking process, this is especially wonderful if you have children (and let go of the fact there maybe more mess than usual). The more love involved, the better a meal will taste.

- ♥ Always **sit down** to eat at a table. Sitting down gets you grounded and helps you to relax.

- ♥ **Look up and switch off**. Turn off the TV, the radio or any mobile devices and engage with those around you at the dinner table. If eating alone, relish the stillness, enjoy the peace, and silence and reflect of the day that has past.

- ♥ Take a mouthful of food then put your cutlery down and **chew slowly**. Enjoy every single mouthful as this is the first stimulating phase in getting your digestion working well.

CHILDREN LOVING VEGETABLES

Yes this does exist! Without the bribes, fights and stress. A simple holistic approach to transform your child/ren from picking out any visible signs of vegetables (especially the green ones), to devouring all varieties in their brightly coloured forms either raw or cooked can be achieved.

My 3 simple steps to family mealtime success:

- ♥ **Get them cooking.** Educate your child/ren and get them involved in the cooking process from as young as possible. Talk about what meals they love; let them pick out recipes from cookbooks or magazines; when shopping, allow them to select, sniff and feel. Enable them to stand beside you and help prepare food, tasting as they go.

- ♥ **Talk fun food health facts.** From the moment our children were eating solids I spoke to them, and then with them as they grew, about the benefits of wholefoods. Not in a dictated way, just in general terms like "wow can you see when mummy slices the carrot into circles it looks like an eye? Carrots are so clever, when you eat them they actually help you to see so you can read your favourite books better".

- ♥ **Get positive backup.** Let's face it, your child/ren will get drummed out by your constant natter about eating vegetales so enlist backup. Have a person that your child admires talk to them. It could be their father, grandma or grandpa, an older cousin, neighbourhood friend, aunt or uncle – the idea here is that it is not coming from you. My husband once used "when daddy eats green vegetables I have so much more energy to run fast and you will too, which means lots of extra playtime with your friends at daycare – how much fun is that!"

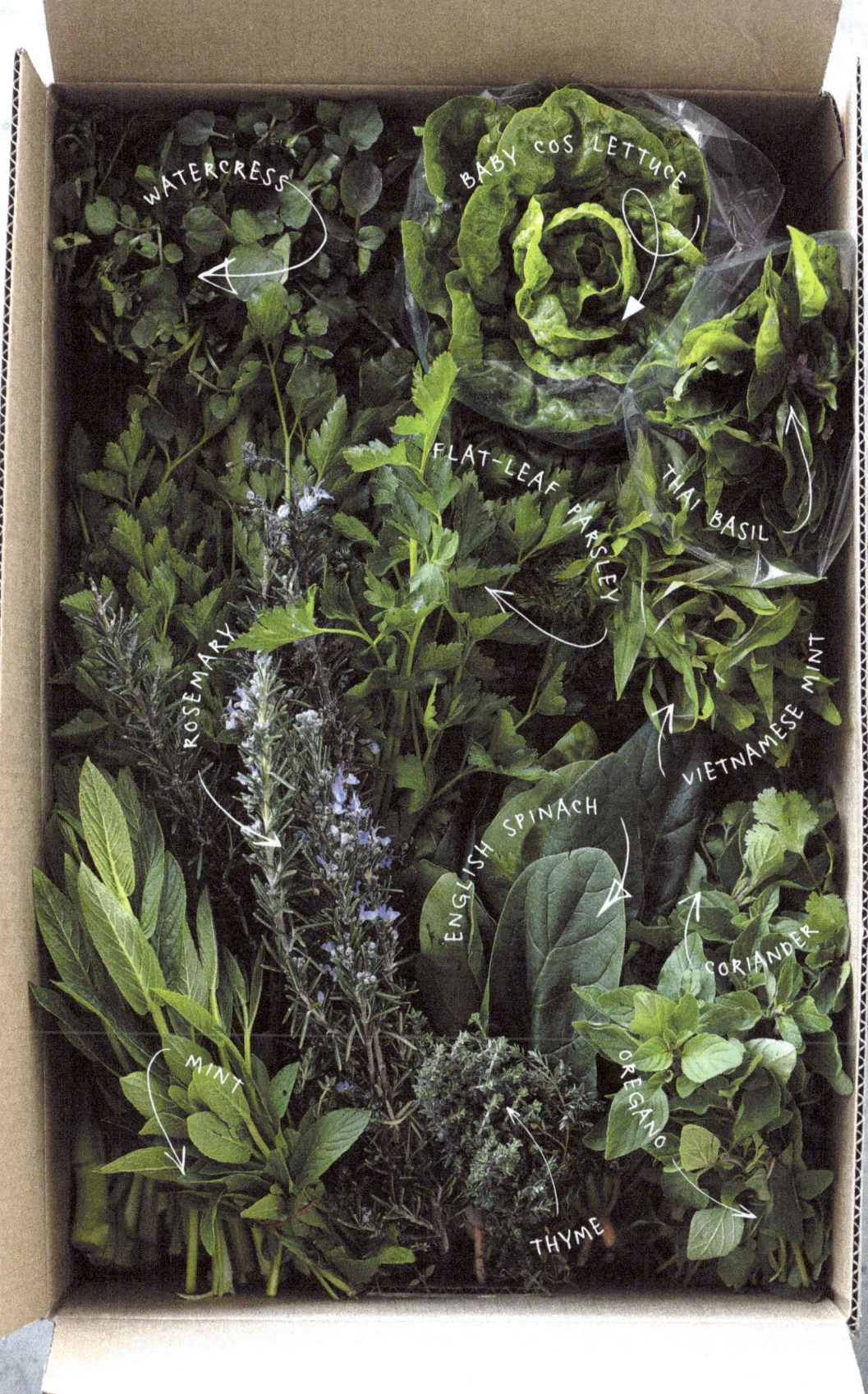

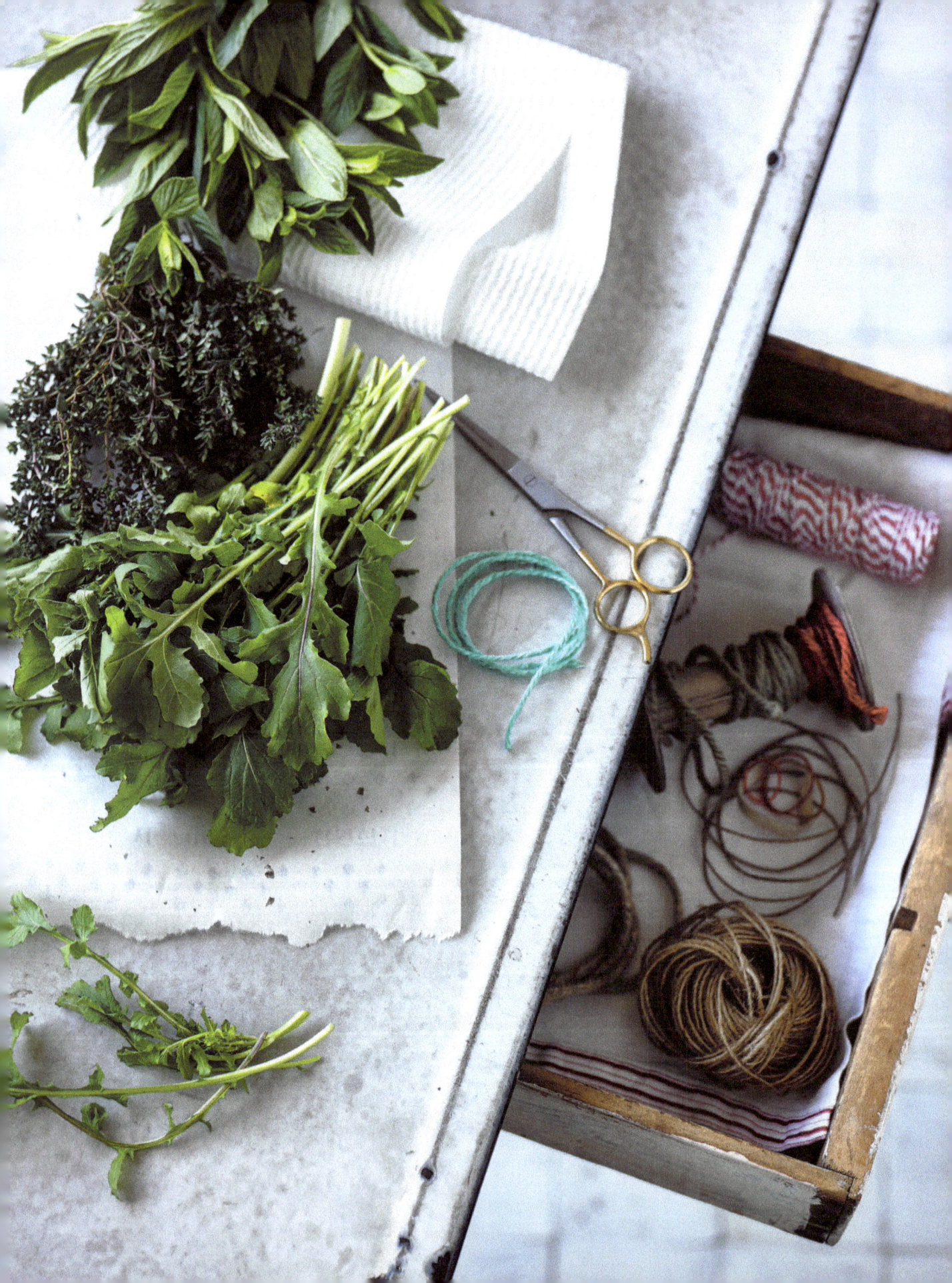

About My Recipes

SERVING SIZES ARE FOR 6

I have developed all my recipes to serve 6 because households have expanded. Many of my friends are having 3+ children these days and even though we are a complete family of 4, I do always like to have some leftovers from dinner as they are great for either breakfast or lunch the following day.

BATCH COOKING

I love finding a day every few weeks where I spend the time making big batches of my recipes, then freezing them into portions. It really does save a lot of stress and time in the kitchen when you have those crazy busy weeks and are able to just grab and re-heat something from the freezer. You will find that the majority of the recipes in the cookbook are freezer-friendly (FF) and can easily be doubled or tripled. For those who are in a single household, simply cook the recipes as directed and freeze into single portions.

HERB BUNCHES

You will notice in my recipes that I refer to fresh herb bunches as either 'small' or 'large'. I find that if you need to purchase herbs from a large-scale supermarket their bunches of herbs are quite smaller than those you can purchase from a greengrocer or farmers market. The truth is, it doesn't really matter. Add as little or as much as you like – I love using large amounts in all of my cooking for added flavour and nutrition.

VEGETABLE & FRUIT PREPARATION

I always leave the skins on my vegetables and fruit (unless otherwise stated in the recipe ingredient list) and just give them a really good scrub under running water before using. Firstly, it saves valuable food preparation time but more importantly it's because the skins of vegetables and fruit can be great sources of beneficial phytochemicals, antioxidants and good sources of insoluble fibre.

KEEP VEGETABLE TRIMMINGS

Keep all of your other vegetable trimmings and use them to make delicious homemade stock. Simply give them a good rinse under cold running water then place into a large freezer-safe resealable bag and freeze. Keep adding trimmings to the bag until it is completely filled, then add to your stockpot along with your chosen poultry, fish or meat bones when making stock.

RECIPE SYMBOLS

You will find each recipe features symbols so you can quickly identify what will suit you and your family's needs best. Maybe you or someone in your household has a food sensitivity, intolerance, allergy or perhaps you are just looking for a recipe that is freezer-friendly.

HERE ARE WHAT MY RECIPE SYMBOLS LOOK LIKE

DF – dairy-free

GRF – grain-free

NF – nut-free

RSF – refined sugar-free

P – paleo

V – vegetarian

VG – vegan

FF – freezer-friendly

RECIPE MEASUREMENTS

I use Standard Metric Measures and all measures are level.

1 teaspoon = 5ml

1 tablespoon = 20ml

1 cup = 250ml

OVEN TEMPERATURES

Oven temperatures are given for conventional ovens along with a fan-forced (convection) oven temperature reduction of 20°C. Not all ovens are created equal so it is best to always refer to your manufacturer's handbook for recommendations.

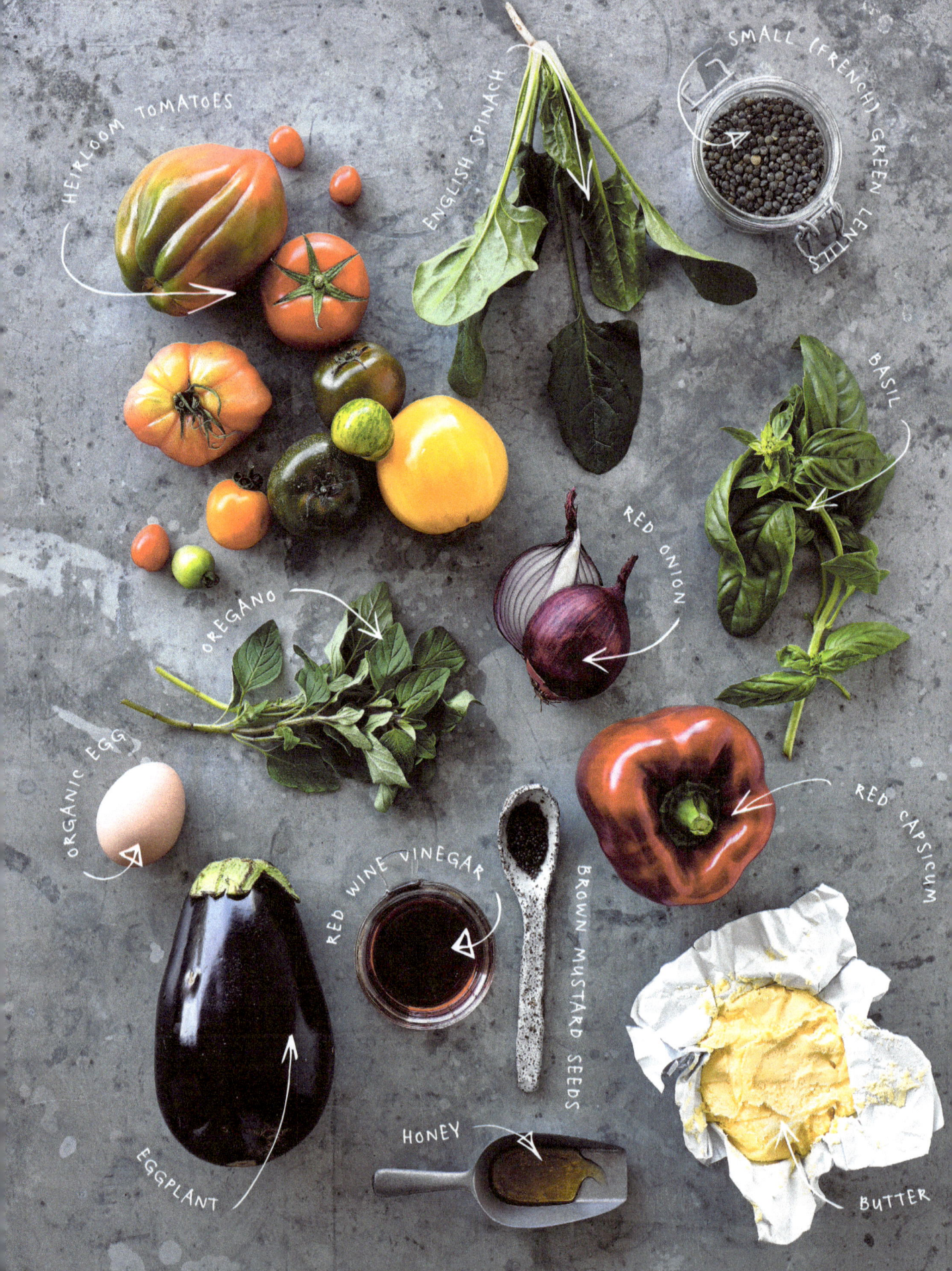

tomato sauce

Basic Tomato Sauce / *25*
Tomato & Peach Chutney / *26*
Lentil Pasta Sauce / *29*
Buttery Chicken Curry / *30*
Anytime Eggs / *33*

ALL ABOUT TOMATO SAUCE

One of the best homemade versions of a classic store-bought product that I cook all year round. It is so versatile and delicious — I use my recipe for Tomato Sauce in any recipe that requires either canned tomatoes or tomato passata. Our family also enjoy using it in place of store bought tomato ketchup. You will get a wider variety of delicious tomatoes through the summer months to make Tomato Sauce. In winter months try using a sweet variety of cherry tomatoes to add the extra flavour needed.

♥ When tomatoes are in season, do this

Tomatoes are at their best in summer months, so if you have the time why not buy bulk when they are cheap, cook Tomato Sauce, then freeze into easy grab portions. I like to do 2-cup measurements into freezer-safe resealable bags, then lay them flat, stack and freeze. The Tomato Sauce will keep for 6 months in the freezer and because you freeze the portions flat, they don't take long to defrost in the fridge.

♥ Save time

Prepare your Tomato Sauce ahead of time, as mentioned above, or make and store in an airtight container in the fridge for up to 5 days. This way, when you go to cook the recipe versions your overall cooking time will be minimal.

♥ Types of tomatoes to use

I always use a wide variety of tomatoes when making my sauce, simply because I like how you can vary the flavour and colour. If you use more of the orange and yellow heirloom varieties the colour of your sauce will not be as red. If you use sweeter cherry tomatoes your sauce will obviously taste a lot sweeter and be a richer red colour. It is really up to you, produce availability and also what you enjoy eating the most. You can choose from heirloom varieties, roma, cherry and vine-ripened, to name a few.

♥ Why I use my Tomato Sauce in place of canned tomatoes

It has been shown that there are significant levels of bisphenol A (BPA) in canned foods. BPA is used in the lacquer lining of canned products and just like in plastic products, this toxic chemical can leach into the foods contained within these containers. Since BPA is an endocrine disruptor (interferes with the endocrine or hormonal system), it has been associated with obesity, breast and prostate cancers and behavioural problems.

♥ Sterilising jars

Wash your chosen jars in hot soapy water, then rinse in hot running water. Place them in a low oven (110°C/90°C fan-forced) for 20 minutes or until completely dry.

♥ Storing

Un-opened jars will keep for 6 months when stored in a cool, dark place. Opened refrigerated jars will keep for 1 week.

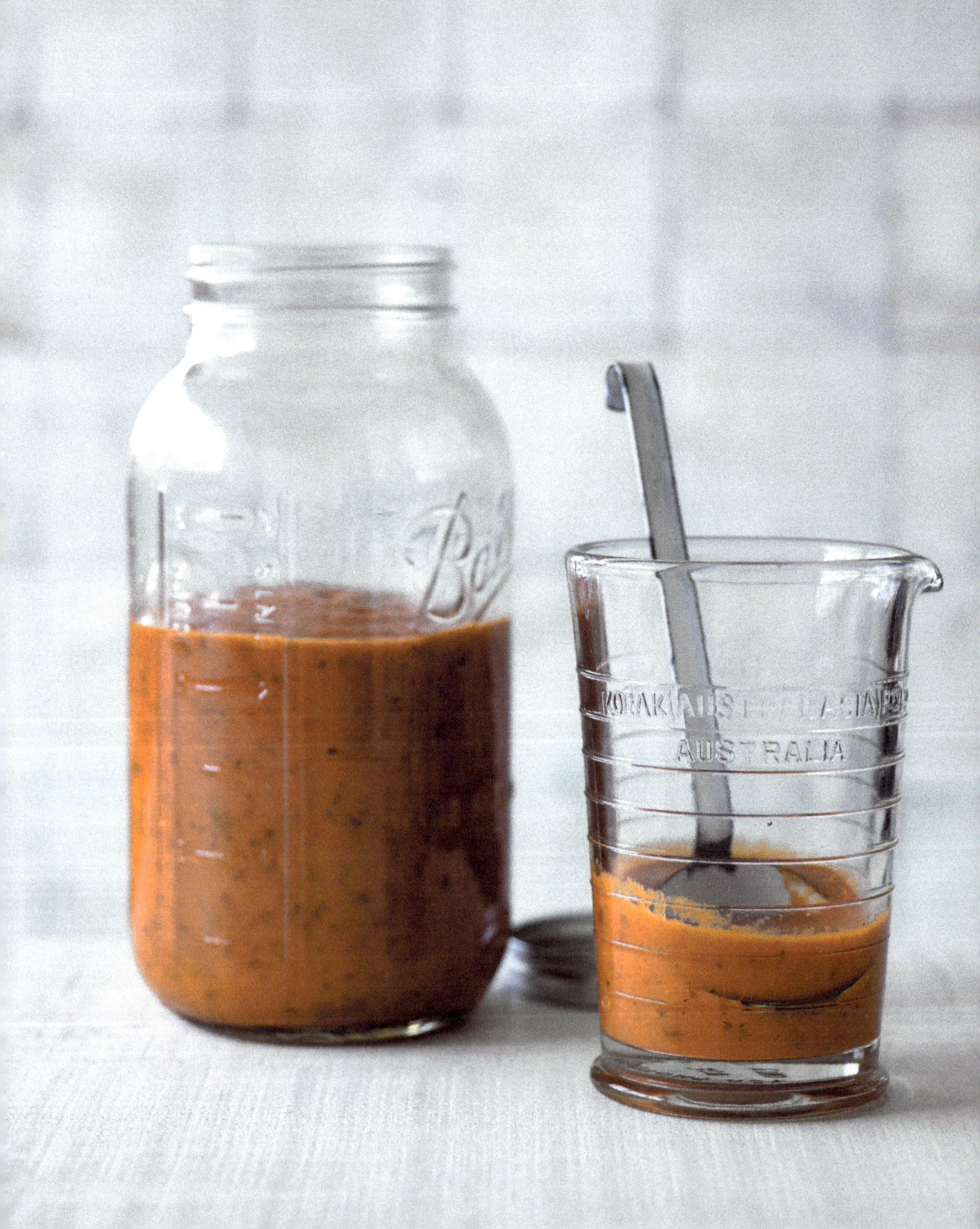

Basic Tomato Sauce

Time to prepare: 20 minutes
Time to cook: 45 minutes + 20 minutes to cool

1. Preheat a large, heavy-based saucepan over a low-medium heat. Add your butter and swirl the pan occasionally until it melts. Stir in your onion and cook, stirring occasionally, for 15 minutes. You want the onion to become very soft and translucent but not to colour too much.

2. Add your tomato and cook, covered and stirring occasionally, for 20 minutes. You want the tomatoes to slowly collapse, becoming soft and releasing all of their natural juice.

3. Stir in all of your remaining ingredients and cook, covered and stirring occasionally, for 10 minutes or until the sauce looks rich in colour and thickens ever so slightly. Season with a little sea salt, then allow your tomato mixture to cool in the pan for 20 minutes.

4. Transfer your tomato mixture to an upright blender and process until smooth. Use your tomato sauce straight away or pour into an airtight container and store in the fridge for up to 5 days.

MAKES: 4 CUPS (1 LITRE)

50g butter
1 red onion, peeled and chopped
1 kg tomatoes, roughly chopped
1 tablespoon red wine vinegar
2 teaspoons honey
½ small bunch fresh basil, leaves picked
1 small bunch fresh oregano, leaves picked

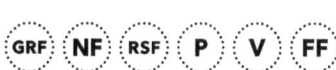

RECIPE SWITCH UP

Add more vegetables – reduce down tomato quantity to 600g and add an additional 500g worth of any vegetables in season. Try parsnip, red cabbage, swede, sweet potato, celery, carrot or zucchini ... Great for fooling little ones.

Tomato & Peach Chutney

Time to prepare: 25 minutes
Time to cook: 1 hour 25 minutes + 20 minutes to cool

MAKES 6 CUPS (1.5 LITRES)

50g butter
1 red onion, peeled and chopped
1 kg tomatoes, roughly chopped
1 tablespoon red wine vinegar
2 teaspoons honey
½ small bunch fresh basil, leaves picked
1 small bunch fresh oregano, leaves picked
⅓ cup 100% maple syrup
4 ripe peaches, stones removed and chopped
3cm piece fresh ginger, peeled and finely grated
1 tablespoon brown mustard seeds

1. Preheat a large, heavy-based saucepan over a low-medium heat. Add your butter and swirl the pan occasionally until it melts. Stir in your onion and cook, stirring occasionally, for 15 minutes. You want the onion to become very soft and translucent but not to colour too much.

2. Add your tomato and cook, covered and stirring occasionally, for 20 minutes. You want the tomatoes to slowly collapse, becoming soft and releasing all of their natural juice.

3. Stir in your vinegar, honey, basil and oregano and cook, covered and stirring occasionally, for 10 minutes or until the sauce looks rich in colour and thickens ever so slightly. Season with a little sea salt, then allow your tomato mixture to cool in the pan for 20 minutes.

4. Transfer your tomato mixture to an upright blender and process until smooth.

5. Pour your tomato sauce back into the same saucepan and place over a medium heat. Stir in your syrup, peach, ginger and mustard seeds and cook, partially covered and stirring occasionally (it tends to catch a little on the base so keep a close eye), for 40 minutes or until the mixture has reduced and is thick. Spoon hot chutney into sterilised jars (see tip pg 23) and secure lids. Cool to room temperature. Serve or store.

RECIPE SWITCH UP

In the summer months you can use any stonefruit that is available in place of the peach and in the winter months you can use apple or pear.

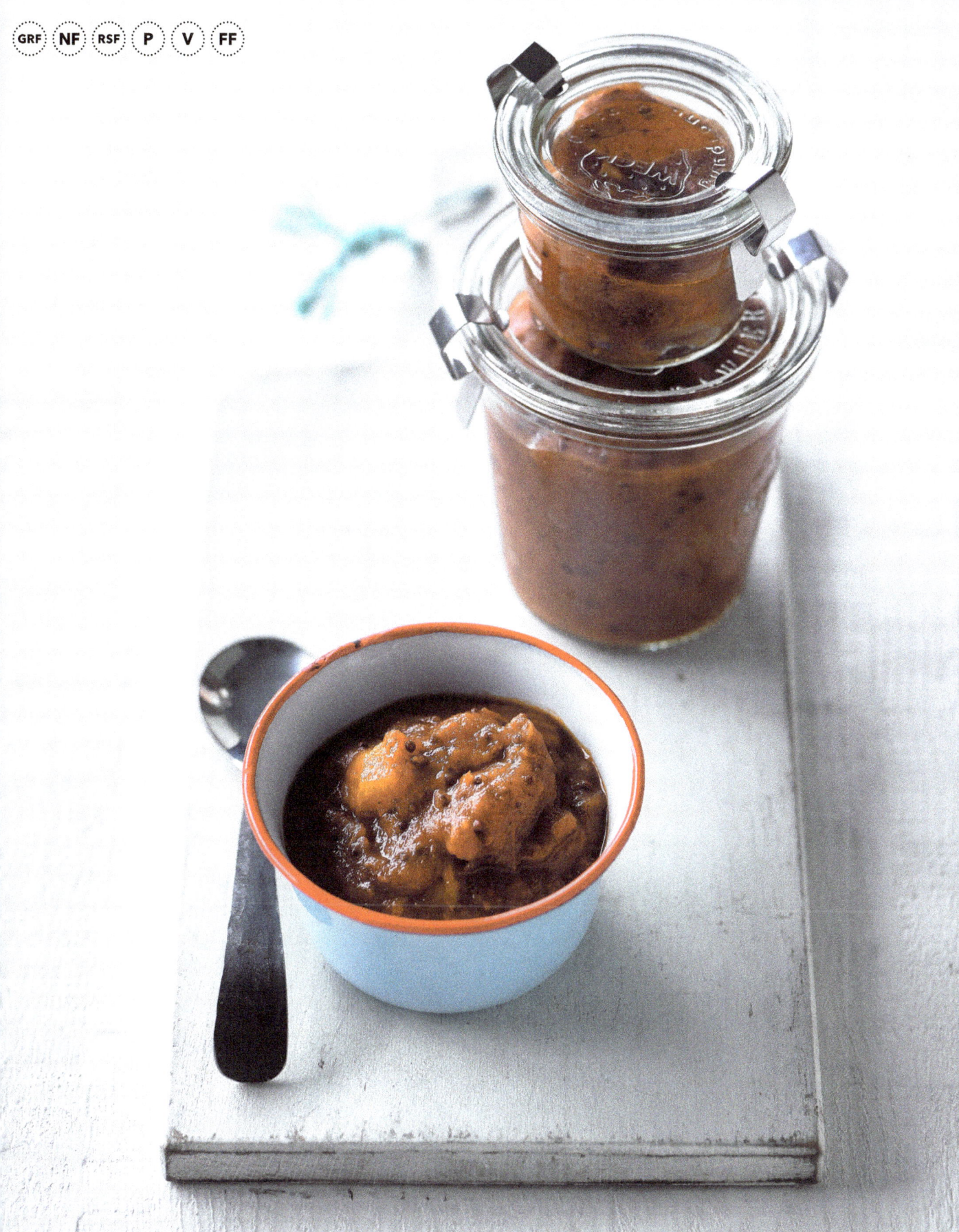

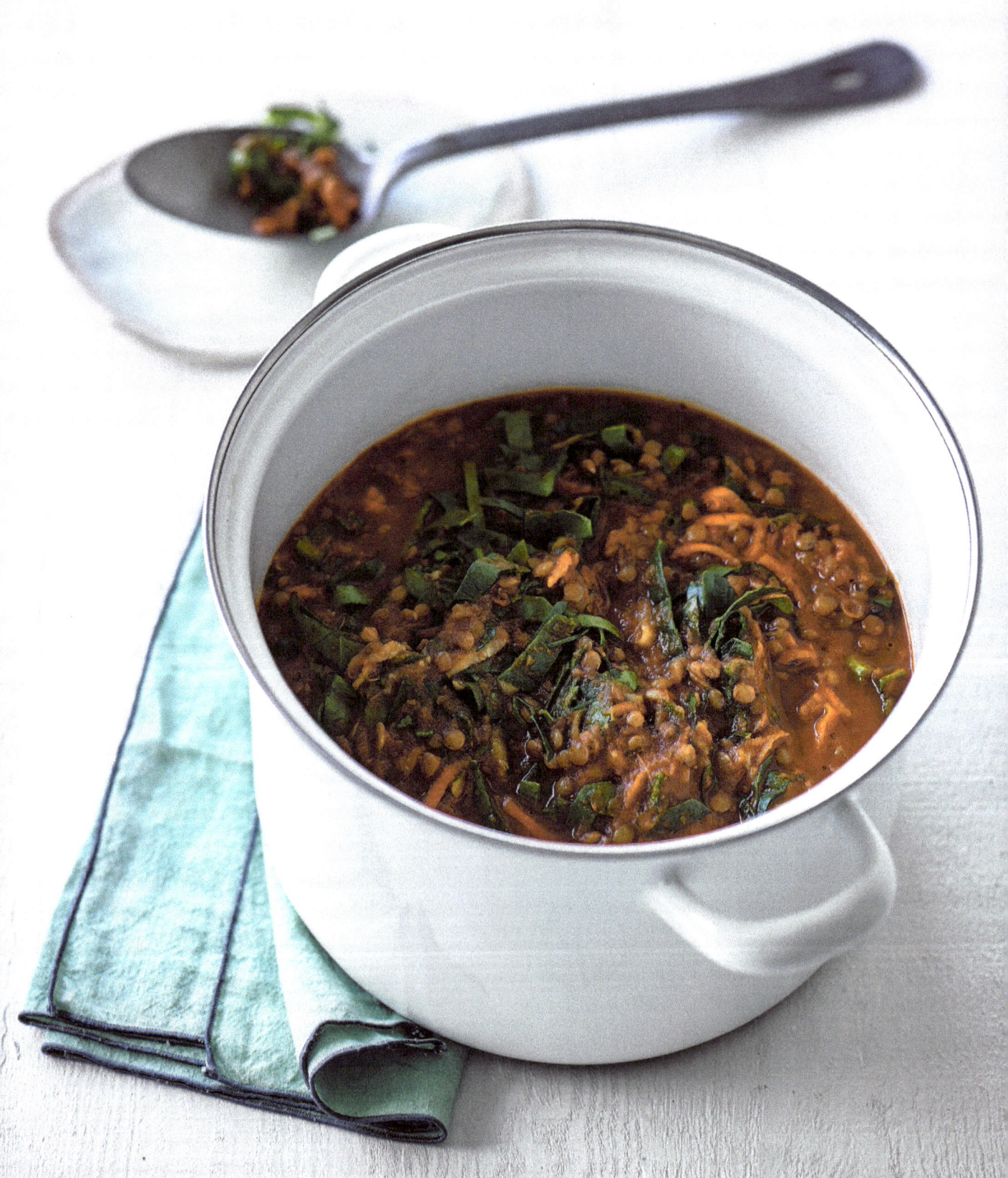

Lentil Pasta Sauce

Time to prepare: 25 minutes
Time to cook: 45 minutes + 20 minutes to cool

1. Preheat a large, heavy-based saucepan over a low-medium heat. Add your butter and swirl the pan occasionally until it melts. Stir in your onion and cook, stirring occasionally, for 15 minutes. You want the onion to become very soft and translucent but not to colour too much.

2. Add your tomato and cook, covered and stirring occasionally, for 20 minutes. You want the tomatoes to slowly collapse, becoming soft and releasing all of their natural juice.

3. Stir in your vinegar, honey, basil and oregano and cook, covered and stirring occasionally, for 10 minutes or until the sauce looks rich in colour and thickens ever so slightly. Season with a little sea salt, then allow your tomato mixture to cool in the pan for 20 minutes.

4. Transfer your tomato mixture to an upright blender and process until smooth.

5. Pour your tomato sauce back into the same saucepan and place over a medium heat. Stir in your lentils, carrot, zucchini and 3 cups (750ml) water and simmer, covered and stirring occasionally, for 30 minutes or until your lentils are tender. Stir in your spinach until just wilted. Season with sea salt and freshly ground black pepper. Serve.

SERVES: 6

50g butter
1 red onion, peeled and chopped
1 kg tomatoes, roughly chopped
1 tablespoon red wine vinegar
2 teaspoons honey
½ small bunch fresh basil, leaves picked
1 small bunch fresh oregano, leaves picked
1 cup dried small (French) green lentils
1 large carrot, coarsely grated
1 large zucchini, coarsely grated
1 bunch English spinach, leaves washed and shredded

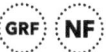

Buttery Chicken Curry

Time to prepare: 30 minutes
Time to cook: 1 hour 5 minutes + 20 minutes to rest

1. Make the Chicken Spice Mix first by combining all of your ingredients together in a large bowl, cover and place in the fridge to marinate while you prepare the rest of the meal (or up to 2 days if you have the time).

2. Preheat a large, heavy-based saucepan over a low-medium heat. Add your butter and swirl the pan occasionally until it melts. Stir in your onion and cook, stirring occasionally, for 15 minutes. You want the onion to become very soft and translucent but not to colour too much.

3. Add your tomato and cook, covered and stirring occasionally, for 20 minutes. You want the tomatoes to slowly collapse, becoming soft and releasing all of their natural juice.

4. Stir in all of your remaining ingredients and cook, covered and stirring occasionally, for 10 minutes or until the sauce looks rich in colour and thickens ever so slightly. Season with a little sea salt, then allow your tomato mixture to cool in the pan for 20 minutes.

5. Transfer your tomato mixture to an upright blender and process until smooth.

6. Reheat the same pan over medium heat. Add half of your extra butter and the marinated chicken mixture, then cook, stirring, for 2 minutes or until fragrant.

7. Add tomato sauce and cook, partially covered and stirring occasionally, for 20 minutes or until chicken has cooked. Stir in your remaining extra butter until melted. Serve.

SERVES: 6

50g butter, plus 100g extra
1 red onion, peeled and chopped
1 kg tomatoes, roughly chopped
1 tablespoon red wine vinegar
2 teaspoons honey
½ small bunch fresh basil, leaves picked
1 small bunch fresh oregano, leaves picked

CHICKEN SPICE MIX

6 chicken thigh fillets, thinly sliced
1 tablespoon garam masala
1 tablespoon ground coriander
1 tablespoon ground cumin
1 teaspoon dried chilli flakes or sweet paprika
3cm piece fresh ginger, peeled and finely grated
2 cloves garlic, peeled and crushed

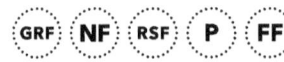

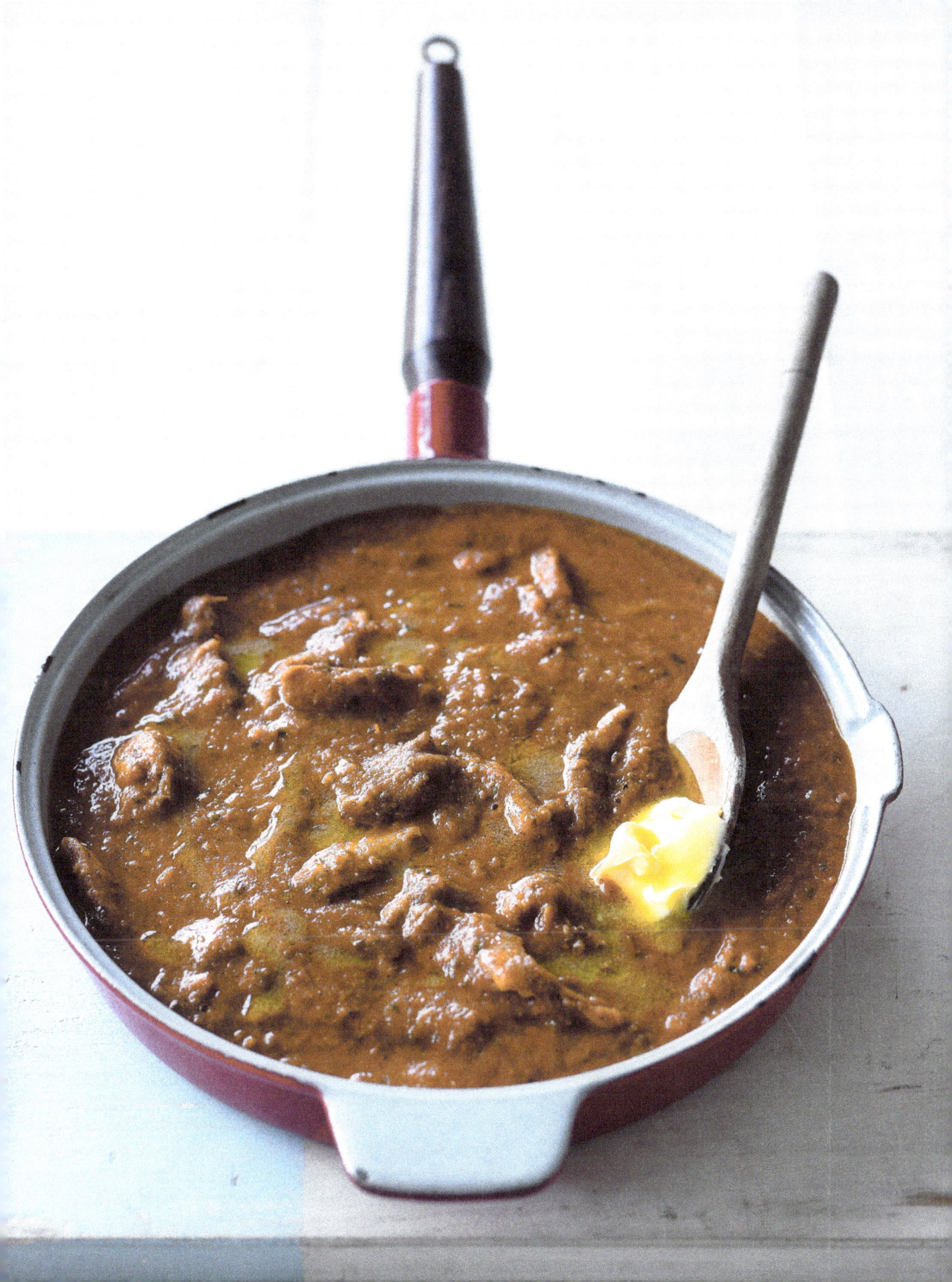

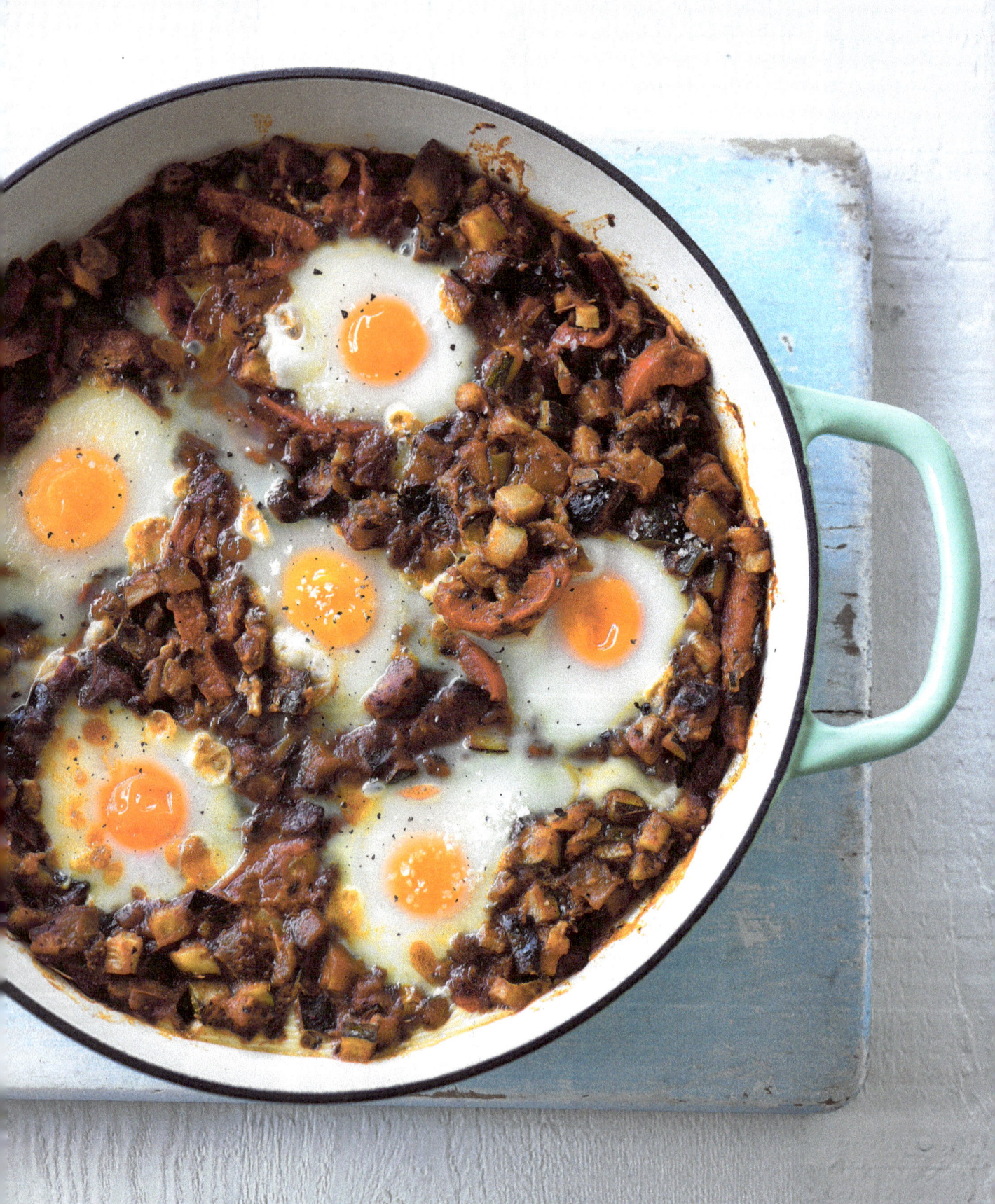

Anytime Eggs

Time to prepare: 35 minutes
Time to cook: 1 hour 13 minutes + 20 minutes to rest

1. Preheat a large, heavy-based saucepan over a low-medium heat. Add half your butter and allow to melt. Stir in your onion and cook, stirring occasionally, for 15 minutes. You want the onion to become very soft but not colour too much.

2. Add tomato and cook, cover and stir occasionally, for 20 minutes. You want them to slowly collapse, becoming soft and releasing all of their natural juice.

3. Stir in vinegar, honey, basil, oregano and cook, covered and stirring occasionally, for 10 minutes or until sauce looks rich and thickens slightly. Season with sea salt, then allow mixture to cool in pan for 20 minutes.

4. Meanwhile, preheat your oven to 180°C/160°C fan-forced.

5. Transfer tomato mixture to an upright blender and process until smooth.

6. Heat a large, deep oven-proof frying pan over a medium heat. Add remaining butter, eggplant, zucchini, capsicum and smoked paprika and cook, stirring occasionally, for 15 minutes or until very soft. Stir in tomato sauce and cook, stirring for 5 minutes or until sauce reduces and thickens.

7. Use the back of a large spoon to make 6 deep indents in tomato mixture. Crack an egg into each indent, then bake for 8 minutes or until egg whites have set and yolks still soft. Season with freshly ground black pepper. Serve.

SERVES: 6

50g butter
1 small red onion, peeled and chopped
500g tomatoes, roughly chopped
2 teaspoons red wine vinegar
1 teaspoon honey
½ small bunch fresh basil, leaves picked
1 small bunch fresh oregano, leaves picked
1 eggplant, chopped
2 zucchini, chopped
1 red capsicum, sliced
3 teaspoons smoked paprika
6 eggs

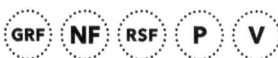

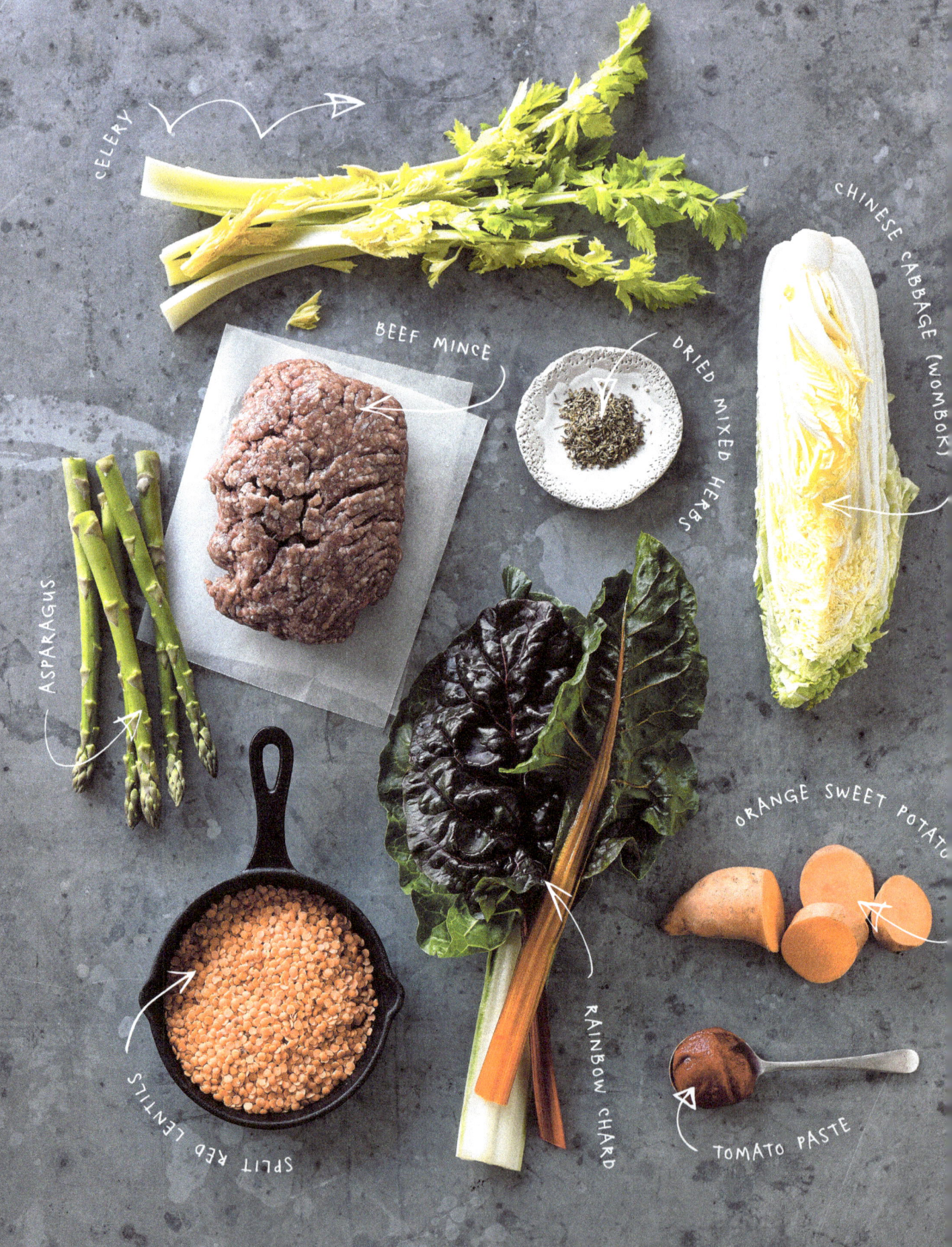

stewp

Basic Stewp / *39*

Almost Meat-free / *40*

Chorizo & Chilli / *43*

Spring Chicken / *44*

Asian Pork & Cabbage / *47*

ALL ABOUT STEWP'S

This isn't a type-o, 'stewp' is my little word to describe my all-in-one-pot meal. It's a combination between a stew and a soup. A dish that is super hearty but still contains a little juice so you can enjoy eating it from a large bowl while using a spoon. This meal is made in one large pot and I always add huge volumes of vegetables, as it's a great way to add extra flavour and nutrition, plus use up any number of vegetables you may have lying around in the bottom of the fridge.

♥ Using a heavy-based saucepan

I use a large heavy-based saucepan as I find that the meat will catch to the base to brown but won't actually burn. I also find that there is enough fat in the mince to prevent this from happening too. However, if you prefer to use a lean mince, are a little concerned or don't have a heavy-based saucepan to use then simply add 1 tablespoon of coconut oil to your mince when cooking.

♥ Browning your meat really well

The idea with browning your mince really well for a good 15 minutes and not stirring it too much is that it will create a lovely brown crust on the base of your pan. This is what adds lots of extra flavour and colour to your stewp when cooking so you don't need to use a stock for flavouring the meal.

♥ Freezer-friendly?

Yes! The stewps are all freezer-friendly. Even though sweet potato technically does not freeze well, it is used in such small quantities in the stewps that I find it holds up quite well when defrosted and re-heated.

♥ Tomato paste

Tomato paste is the result of tomatoes that have had their seeds removed and cooked for very long periods of time, it has a delicious concentrated tomato flavour. Be sure to purchase yours from a glass jar vessel and check the labelling to ensure no extra sugars have been added.

♥ Homemade mince

Making your own beef, pork or chicken mince is so easy. Take your favourite cut of meat (with a little fat on it for added flavour), and place into the freezer for 20 minutes. You want the meat muscles to firm up a bit but not to freeze solid. Chop into rough 2cm pieces then place into the bowl of your food processor and process, using the pulse button, until the mixture looks like mince.

♥ Fresh chilli in family meals

Choose either long red or long green varieties of chillies when adding to a family meal, as these are less fiery. To prepare, simply split them in half lengthwise and use a small teaspoon to scrape away any seeds and white membrane. This is were the "heat" of the chilli is contained, so remove, then chop and use as needed. Your child/ren will get the lovely flavour of the chilli but without the heat.

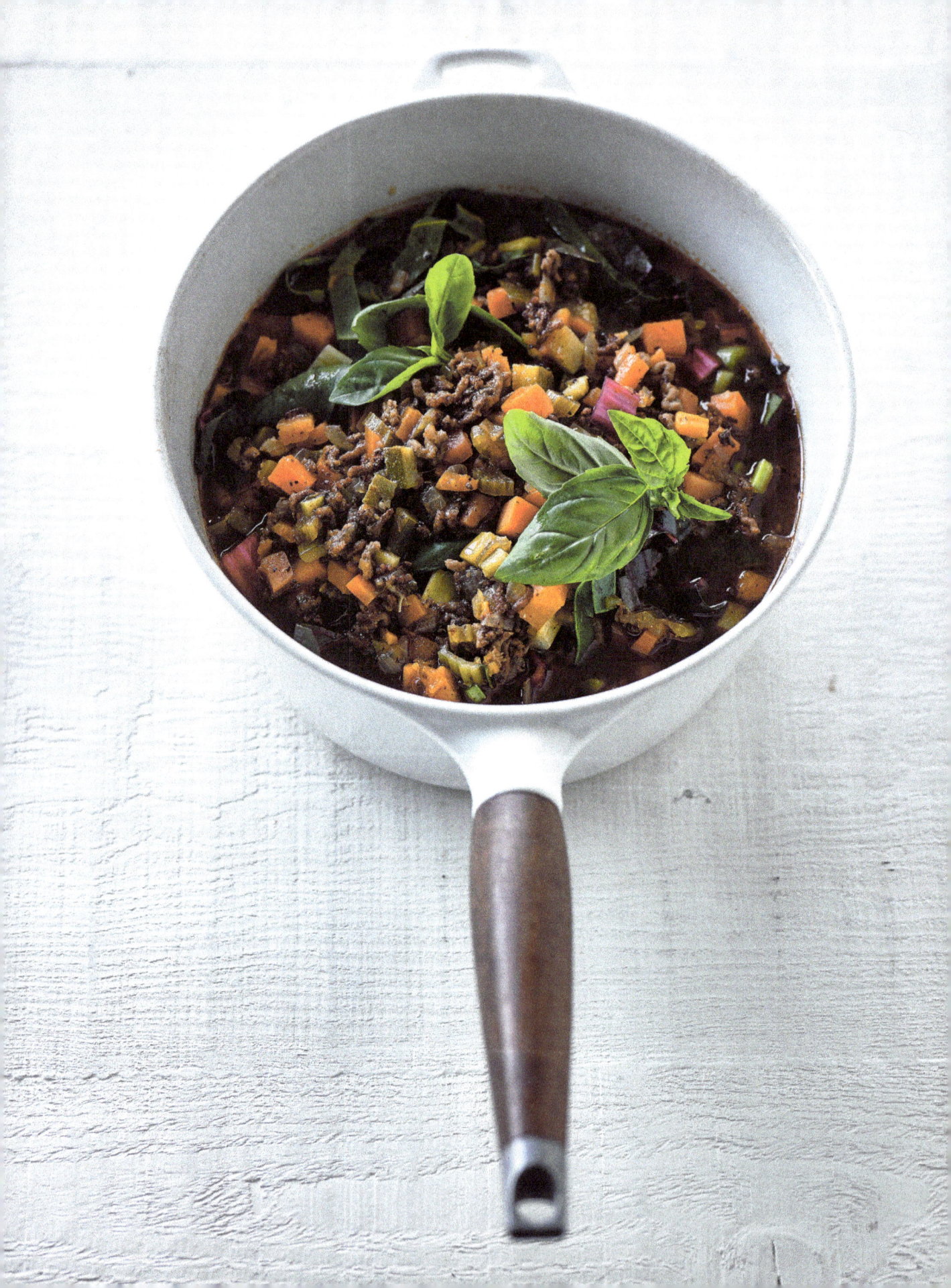

Basic Stewp

Time to prepare: 10 minutes
Time to cook: 45 minutes

1. Preheat a large, heavy-based saucepan over a medium-high heat. Add your mince and don't touch it for 5 minutes to allow it to stick to the base and form a lovely golden crust, then use your spoon to roughly move it around, breaking it into large pieces. Leave it to cook, untouched, for another 5 minutes, before stirring again. Do this process once more, cooking for 5 minutes or until the mince is really lovely and brown and has become dry.

2. Reduce your heat to medium. Add your onion, celery, carrot and zucchini and cook, stirring occasionally, for 15 minutes or until starting to soften. Stir in the tomato paste and dried mixed herbs and cook, stirring, for 5 minutes to cook out the raw flavour of the paste.

3. Stir in your sweet potato and 6 cups (1.5 litres) of boiling water, making sure to scrape the bottom of the pan to release all those lovely beef flavourings. Simmer, partially covered and stirring occasionally, for 15 minutes or until the sweet potato is just tender. Remove the cover and stir in your chard in batches until is just wilts, then stir in the basil. You want to keep a bit of crunch to the chard. Season with sea salt and freshly ground black pepper. Serve the pot straight to the table.

SERVES: 6

500g beef mince
1 large brown onion, peeled and chopped
2 celery stalks, chopped
2 carrots, chopped
2 zucchini, chopped
¼ cup tomato paste
3 teaspoons dried mixed herbs
300g orange sweet potato, chopped
1 bunch rainbow chard, washed and trimmed, then stalks and leaves thinly sliced
1 small bunch fresh basil, leaves picked

RECIPE SWITCH UP

Use 1 bunch of silverbeet in place of the rainbow chard.

HEALTHY MEALS

Almost Meat-free

Time to prepare: 15 minutes
Time to cook: 45 minutes

1. Preheat a large, heavy-based saucepan over a medium-high heat. Add your mince and don't touch it for 5 minutes to allow it to stick to the base and form a lovely golden crust, then use your spoon to roughly move it around, breaking it into large pieces. Leave it to cook, untouched, for another 5 minutes, before stirring again. Do this process once more, cooking for 5 minutes or until the mince is really lovely and brown and has become dry.

2. Reduce your heat to medium. Add your onion, celery, carrot and zucchini and cook, stirring occasionally, for 15 minutes or until starting to soften. Stir in the tomato paste and dried mixed herbs and cook, stirring, for 5 minutes to cook out the raw flavour of the paste.

3. Stir in your sweet potato, lentils and 7 cups (1.75 litres) of boiling water, making sure to scrape the bottom of the pan to release all those lovely beef flavourings. Simmer, partially covered and stirring occasionally, for 15 minutes or until the sweet potato and lentils are just tender. Remove the cover and stir through your parsley and basil. Season with sea salt and freshly ground black pepper. Serve the pot straight to the table.

SERVES: 6

150g beef mince
1 large brown onion, peeled and chopped
2 celery stalks, chopped
2 carrots, chopped
2 zucchini, chopped
¼ cup tomato paste
3 teaspoons dried mixed herbs
300g orange sweet potato, chopped
1 cup dried split red lentils
1 large bunch flat-leaf parsley, stems and leaves chopped
1 small bunch fresh basil, leaves picked

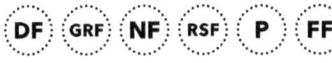

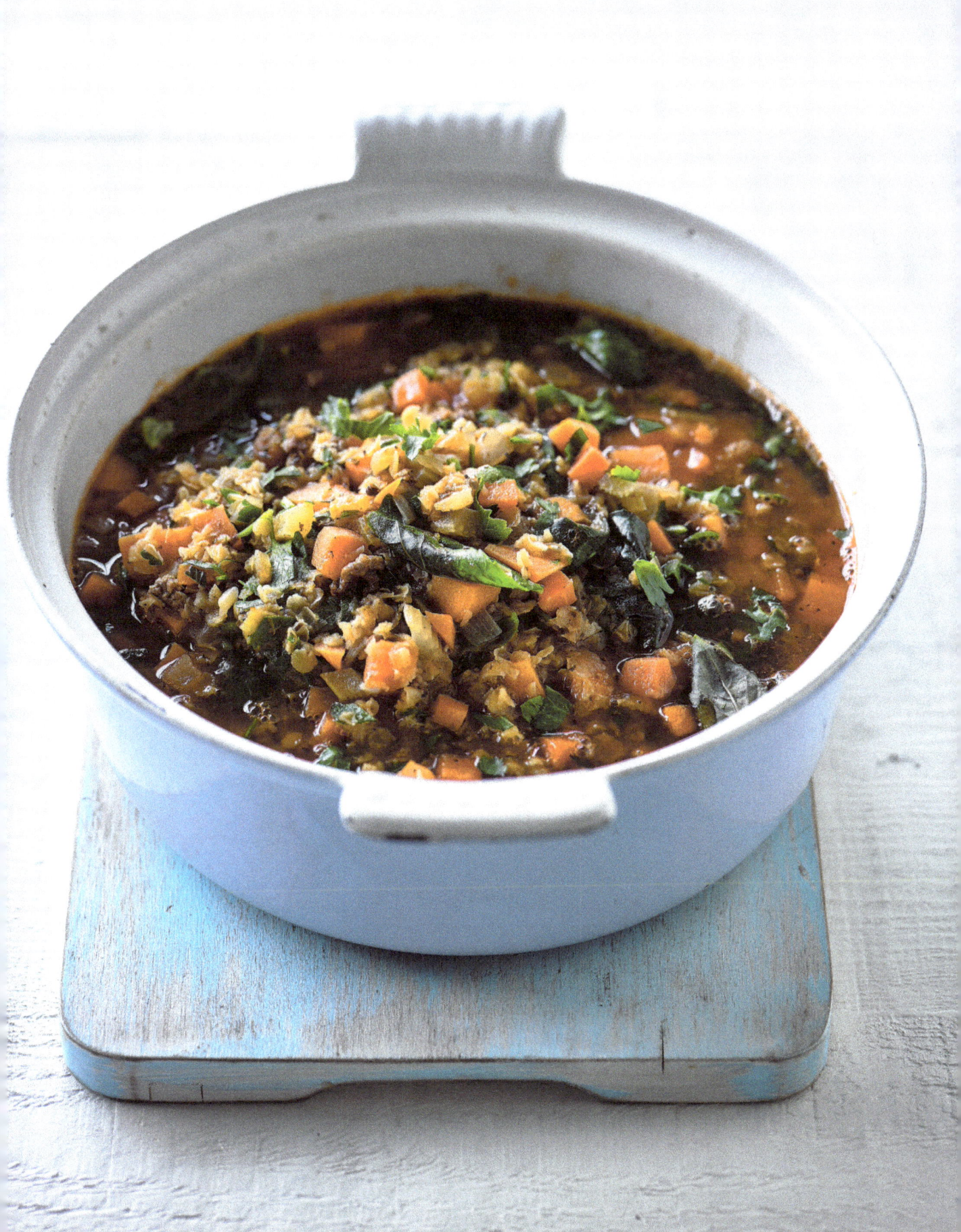

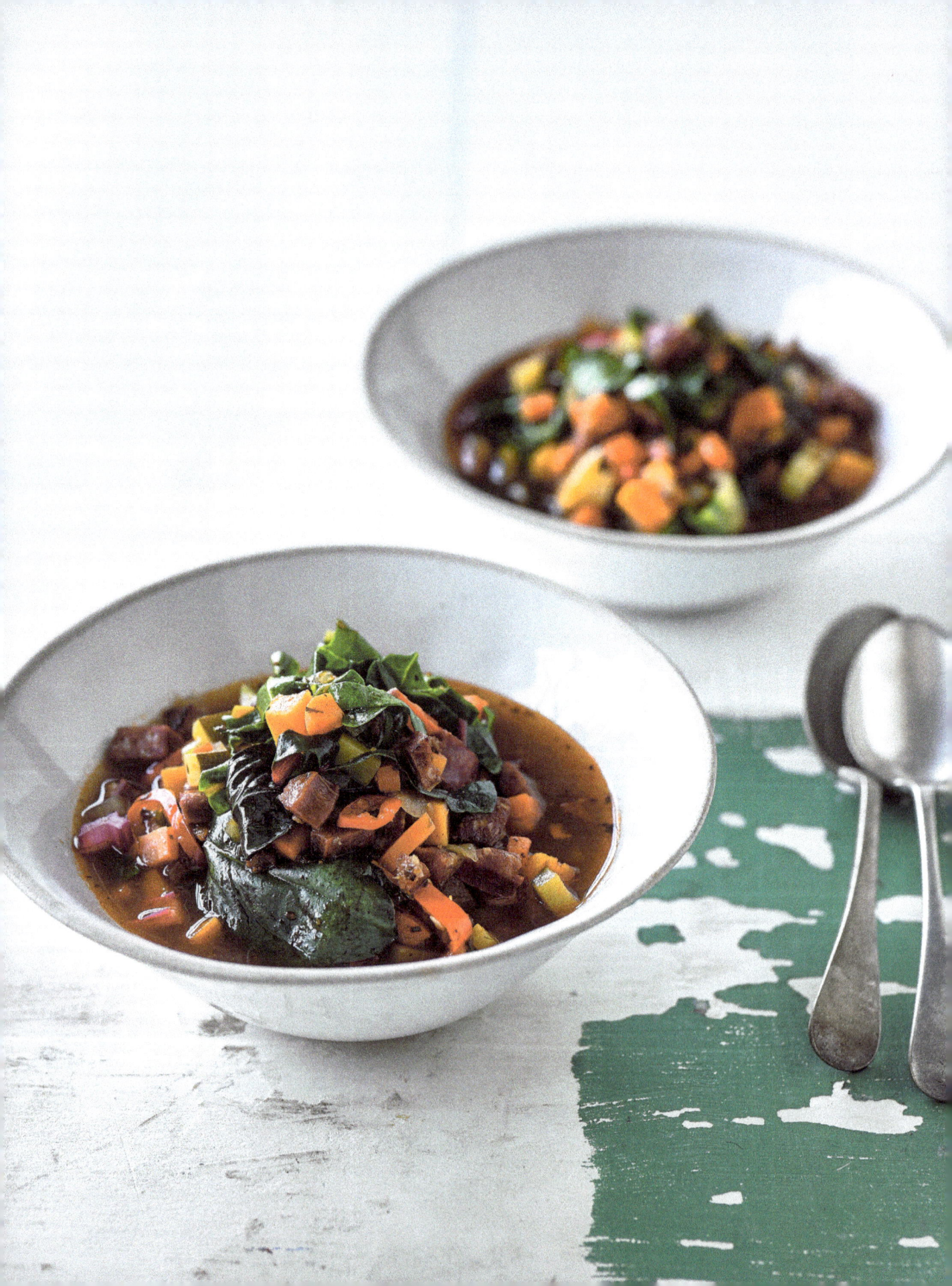

Chorizo & Chilli

Time to prepare: 15 minutes
Time to cook: 45 minutes

1. Preheat a large, heavy-based saucepan over a medium-high heat. Add your mince and chorizo and don't touch it for 5 minutes to allow it to stick to the base and form a lovely golden crust, then use your spoon to roughly move it around, breaking it into large pieces. Leave it to cook, untouched, for another 5 minutes, before stirring again. Do this process once more, cooking for 5 minutes or until the mince is really lovely and brown and has become dry.

2. Reduce your heat to medium. Add your onion, celery, carrot and zucchini and cook, stirring occasionally, for 15 minutes or until starting to soften. Stir in the tomato paste, chilli and dried mixed herbs and cook, stirring, for 5 minutes to cook out the raw flavour of the paste.

3. Stir in your sweet potato and 6 cups (1.5 litres) of boiling water, making sure to scrape the bottom of the pan to release all those lovely beef flavourings. Simmer, partially covered and stirring occasionally, for 15 minutes or until the sweet potato is just tender. Remove the cover and stir in your chard in batches until is just wilts, then stir in the basil. You want to keep a bit of crunch to the chard. Season with sea salt and freshly ground black pepper. Serve.

SERVES: 6

250g beef mince
2 cured chorizo sausages, chopped
1 large brown onion, peeled and chopped
2 celery stalks, chopped
2 carrots, chopped
2 zucchini, chopped
¼ cup tomato paste
2 fresh long red chillies, thinly sliced
3 teaspoons dried mixed herbs
300g orange sweet potato, chopped
1 bunch rainbow chard, washed and trimmed, then stalks and leaves thinly sliced
1 small bunch fresh basil, leaves picked

Spring Chicken

Time to prepare: 15 minutes
Time to cook: 40 minutes

1. Preheat a large, heavy-based saucepan over a medium-high heat. Add your mince and don't touch it for 5 minutes to allow it to stick to the base and form a lovely golden crust, then use your spoon to roughly move it around, breaking it into large pieces. Leave it to cook, untouched, for another 5 minutes or until the mince is really lovely and light brown and has become dry.

2. Reduce your heat to medium. Add your onion, celery, carrot, zucchini and fennel and cook, stirring occasionally, for 15 minutes or until starting to soften. Stir in the dried mixed herbs and cook, stirring, for 1 minute or until fragrant.

3. Stir in your sweet potato and 6 cups (1.5 litres) of boiling water, making sure to scrape the bottom of the pan to release all those lovely beef flavourings. Simmer, partially covered and stirring occasionally, for 15 minutes or until the sweet potato is just tender. Remove the cover and stir in your asparagus, basil, tarragon and spinach until leaves just wilt. You want to keep a bit of crunch to the asparagus. Season with sea salt and freshly ground black pepper. Serve the pot straight to the table.

SERVES: 6

500g chicken mince
1 large brown onion, peeled and chopped
2 celery stalks, chopped
2 carrots, chopped
2 zucchini, chopped
1 fennel, trimmed and sliced
3 teaspoons dried mixed herbs
300g orange sweet potato, chopped
1 bunch asparagus, trimmed and cut into 4cm lengths
1 small bunch fresh basil, leaves picked
1 small bunch fresh tarragon, leaves picked
50g baby spinach leaves

(DF) (GRF) (NF) (RSF) (P) (FF)

RECIPE SWITCH UP

Use baby kale leaves in place of the baby spinach leaves.

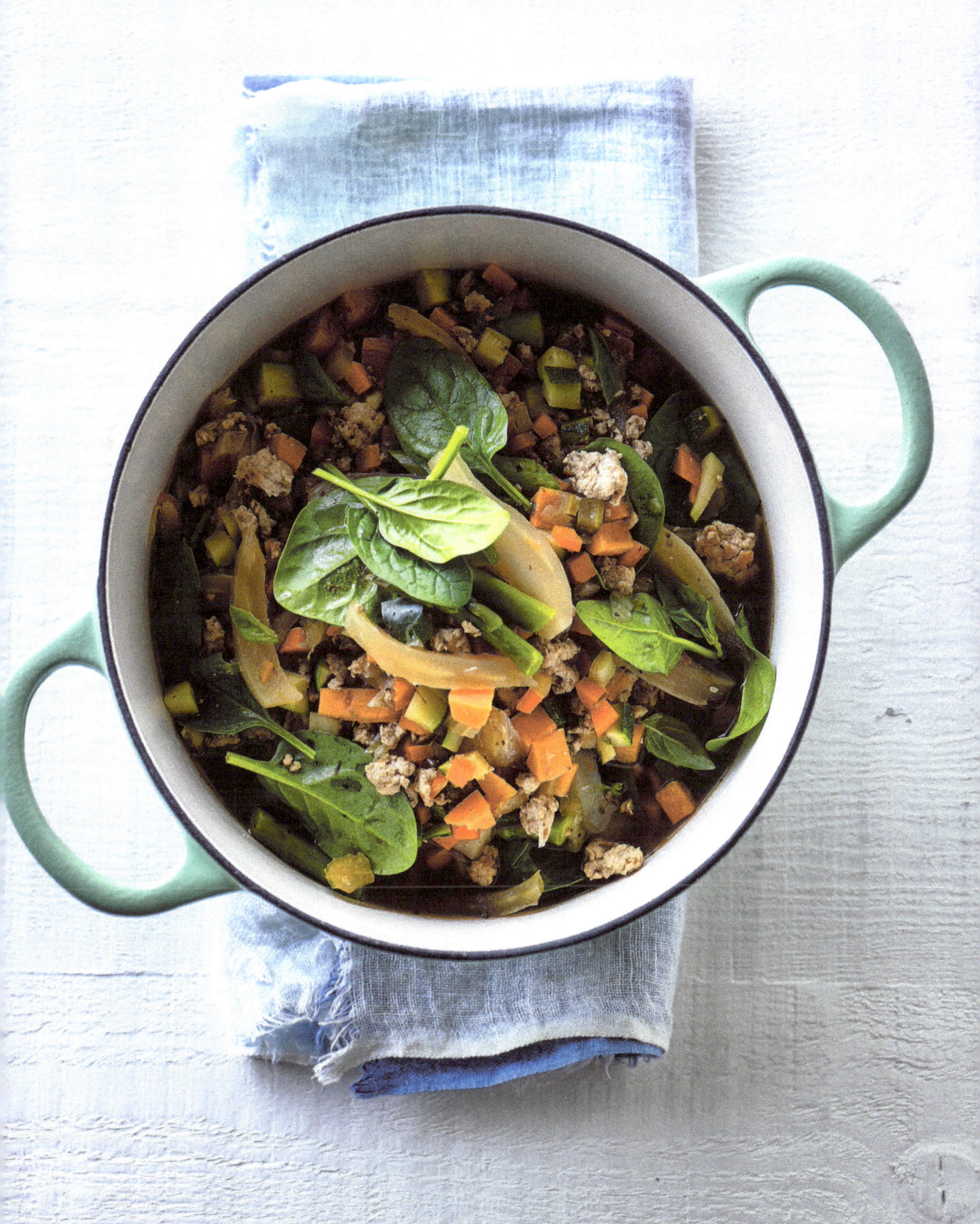

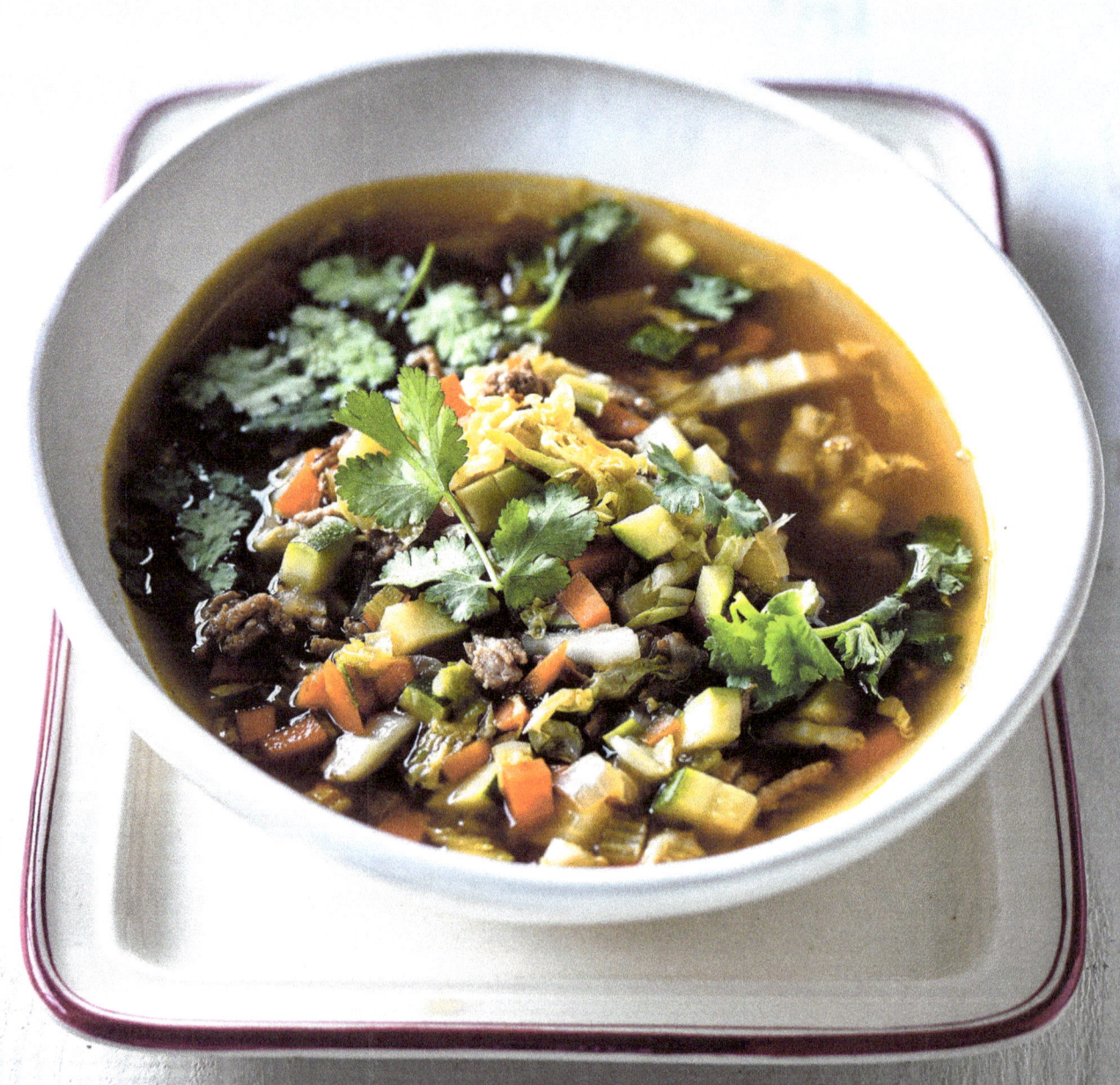

Asian Pork & Cabbage

Time to prepare: 15 minutes
Time to cook: 41 minutes

SERVES: 6

500g pork mince
1 large brown onion, peeled and chopped
2 celery stalks, chopped
2 carrots, chopped
2 zucchini, chopped
2 teaspoons Chinese 5 spice powder
300g orange sweet potato, chopped
2 cups shredded Chinese cabbage (wombok)
1 small bunch fresh basil, leaves picked
1 small bunch fresh coriander, leaves picked

1. Preheat a large, heavy-based saucepan over a medium-high heat. Add your mince and don't touch it for 5 minutes to allow it to stick to the base and form a lovely golden crust, then use your spoon to roughly move it around, breaking it into large pieces. Leave it to cook, untouched, for another 5 minutes or until the mince is really lovely and light brown and has become dry.

2. Reduce your heat to medium. Add your onion, celery, carrot and zucchini and cook, stirring occasionally, for 15 minutes or until starting to soften. Stir in the 5 spice and cook, stirring, for 1 minute or until fragrant.

3. Stir in your sweet potato and 6 cups (1.5 litres) of boiling water, making sure to scrape the bottom of the pan to release all those lovely beef flavourings. Simmer, partially covered and stirring occasionally, for 15 minutes or until the sweet potato is just tender. Remove the cover and stir in your Chinese cabbage until it just wilts, then stir in the basil and coriander. You want to keep a bit of crunch to the cabbage. Season with sea salt and freshly ground black pepper. Serve.

TARRAGON

ORGANIC WHOLE CHICKEN

LEEK

THYME

MIXED BABY CARROTS

BABY BOK CHOY

BABY FENNEL

FENNEL SEEDS

roasting chicken

Basic Roast Chicken / *53*

Pistachio & Herb Stuffed Chicken / *54*

Jerk Chicken / *57*

Steam-roasted Chinese Chicken / *58*

Weeknight Roast Chicken / *61*

ALL ABOUT ROASTING CHICKEN

I think that roasting a chicken for dinner is one of the easiest meals to do. Everything goes in together, pop it in the oven and literally forget about it for 1 hour. If your roasting pan has the space, add a second chicken and then once roasted and cooled, pull off the meat and portion up for lunches over the next 2 days — another simple step to making life just a little bit easier.

Why organic?

In short, they are treated better when reared and as a result they have better flavour and remain really juicy with breast meat that never dries out.

Why you should never wash your raw chicken

You should never wash or rinse your raw chicken under cold running water as this will spread bacteria throughout your kitchen. All you need to do is use disposable kitchen paper towels to pat dry your chicken inside and out.

Safe food handling of raw chicken

- ♥ Place fresh chicken onto a plate, this will help prevent any raw chicken juice spilling throughout your fridge and contaminating other raw foods. Store in your fridge and use within 2 days of purchase.

- ♥ If you froze your chicken after purchasing and need to defrost a frozen chicken, place onto a tray with a high lip, this will help prevent any raw chicken juice spilling throughout your fridge and contaminating other raw foods. Thaw in fridge, never on kitchen bench, overnight.

- Wash your hands thoroughly before and after preparing raw chicken.
- Always use a separate board to prepare raw chicken and wash thoroughly using hot soapy water, along with any utensils used in the preparation.
- Clean surfaces well after preparation.

Resting your roast

It is always important to rest your roast after baking to let the meat relax. The roasting process tightens the meat, trapping all of the natural juices toward the centre of the flesh. On resting, this juice will slowly be reabsorbed back through the flesh as it relaxes making the meat softer on the palette and easier to carve.

Easy guide to carving

Make sure your chicken is facing breast up, remove the leg by pulling away and once it naturally exposes the hip joint (between the breast and the thigh), use your knife to cut through the joint. Pull away the wings and cut through their joint, then slice away the breast meat from the bone.

Don't throw away your roasted chicken carcass

Turn it into chicken stock. Place your carcass into a stockpot and add any vegetable trimmings you have been keeping (see note pg 28), then cover with water. Bring to the boil over a high heat. Once bubbling away reduce it down to a low-medium heat. Use a large slotted spoon to scoop away any frothy impurities that float to the surface and allow to simmer for 1 hour. Strain and discard all of the flavourings then use your stock straight away or cool and store in a large airtight container in the fridge for 1 week or in the freezer for up to 6 months.

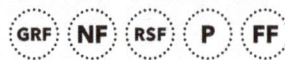

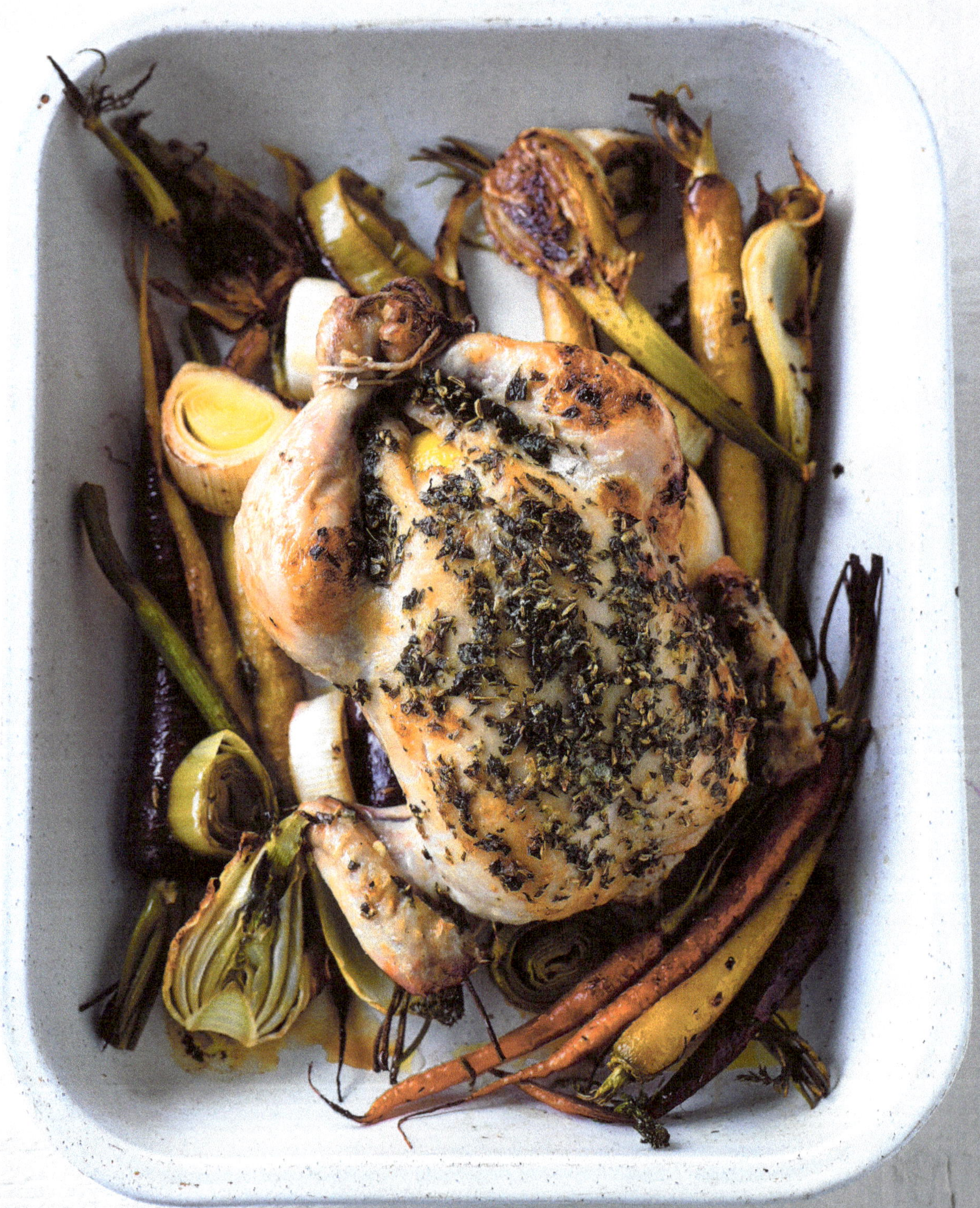

Basic Roast Chicken

Time to prepare: 20 minutes
Time to cook: 1 hour + 15 minutes to rest

1. Preheat your oven for a good 15 minutes to 200°C/180°C fan-forced.

2. Pop your leek, carrot and fennel into a large heavy-based roasting pan. Season with sea salt and freshly ground black pepper.

3. Using kitchen paper towels, pat dry your chicken inside and out, tie legs together, then rest your chicken on top of your vegetables in pan. Season with sea salt and freshly ground black pepper.

4. Stir the softened butter, fennel seeds and tarragon together, then spread the mixture all over the breast area and legs of the chicken. Squeeze the lemon halves all over, then place into chicken cavity. Pour ½ cup of water into the base of the pan (this will help to steam roast the vegetables for you).

5. Roast your chicken for 1 hour. Remove from oven and insert a skewer into the thigh meat to see if the juice runs clear, if it is still tinged pink then return to the oven to roast for another 15 minutes before testing again. Your chicken should have a lovely crisp golden skin and tender moist meat. Once removed from the oven, stand at room temperature lightly covered in foil for 15 minutes to allow the meat to rest. Serve at the table and carve as needed, providing a large spoon for scooping up all the delicious vegetables and pan juices.

SERVES: 6

2 leeks, trimmed, rinsed and thickly sliced
2 bunches mixed baby carrots, trimmed and skins scrubbed
3 baby fennel, trimmed and thickly sliced lengthwise
1.3 kg fresh organic whole chicken
80g butter, at room temperature
2 teaspoons fennel seeds
1 small bunch fresh tarragon, leaves picked and chopped
1 lemon, halved

RECIPE SWITCH UP

- Use 3 carrots, quartered lengthwise, instead of the baby carrots.

- Use either 3 roma tomatoes, halved lengthwise, or 3 large field mushrooms, halved, instead of fennel when not in season.

HEALTHY MEALS

Pistachio & Herb Stuffed Chicken

Time to prepare: 25 minutes
Time to cook: 1 hour + 15 minutes to rest

1. Preheat your oven for a good 15 minutes to 200°C/180°C fan-forced.
2. Pop your leek, carrot and fennel into a large heavy-based roasting pan. Season with sea salt and freshly ground black pepper.
3. Using kitchen paper towels, pat dry your chicken inside and out, tie legs together, then rest your chicken on top of your vegetables in pan. Season with sea salt and freshly ground black pepper.
4. Stir the softened butter, fennel seeds, tarragon, pistachio and thyme together. Using your fingers, gently release the skin from the chicken breast area to create a pocket. Press the butter mixture into the pocket underneath the skin and spread to cover entire breast meat area. Squeeze the lemon halves all over, then place into chicken cavity. Pour ½ cup of water into the base of the pan (this will help to steam roast the vegetables for you).
5. Roast your chicken for 1 hour. Remove from oven and insert a skewer into the thigh meat to see if the juice runs clear, if it is still tinged pink then return to the oven to roast for another 15 minutes before testing again. Your chicken should have a lovely crisp golden skin and tender moist meat. Once removed from the oven, stand at room temperature lightly covered in foil for 15 minutes to allow the meat to rest. Serve at the table and carve as needed, providing a large spoon for scooping up all the delicious vegetables and pan juices.

SERVES: 6

2 leeks, trimmed, rinsed and thickly sliced
2 bunches mixed baby carrots, trimmed and skins scrubbed
3 baby fennel, trimmed and thickly sliced lengthwise
1.3 kg fresh organic whole chicken
80g butter, at room temperature
2 teaspoons fennel seeds
1 small bunch fresh tarragon, leaves picked and chopped
¼ cup pistachio kernels, roasted and finely chopped
½ bunch fresh thyme, leaves picked
1 lemon, halved

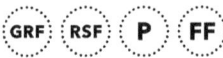

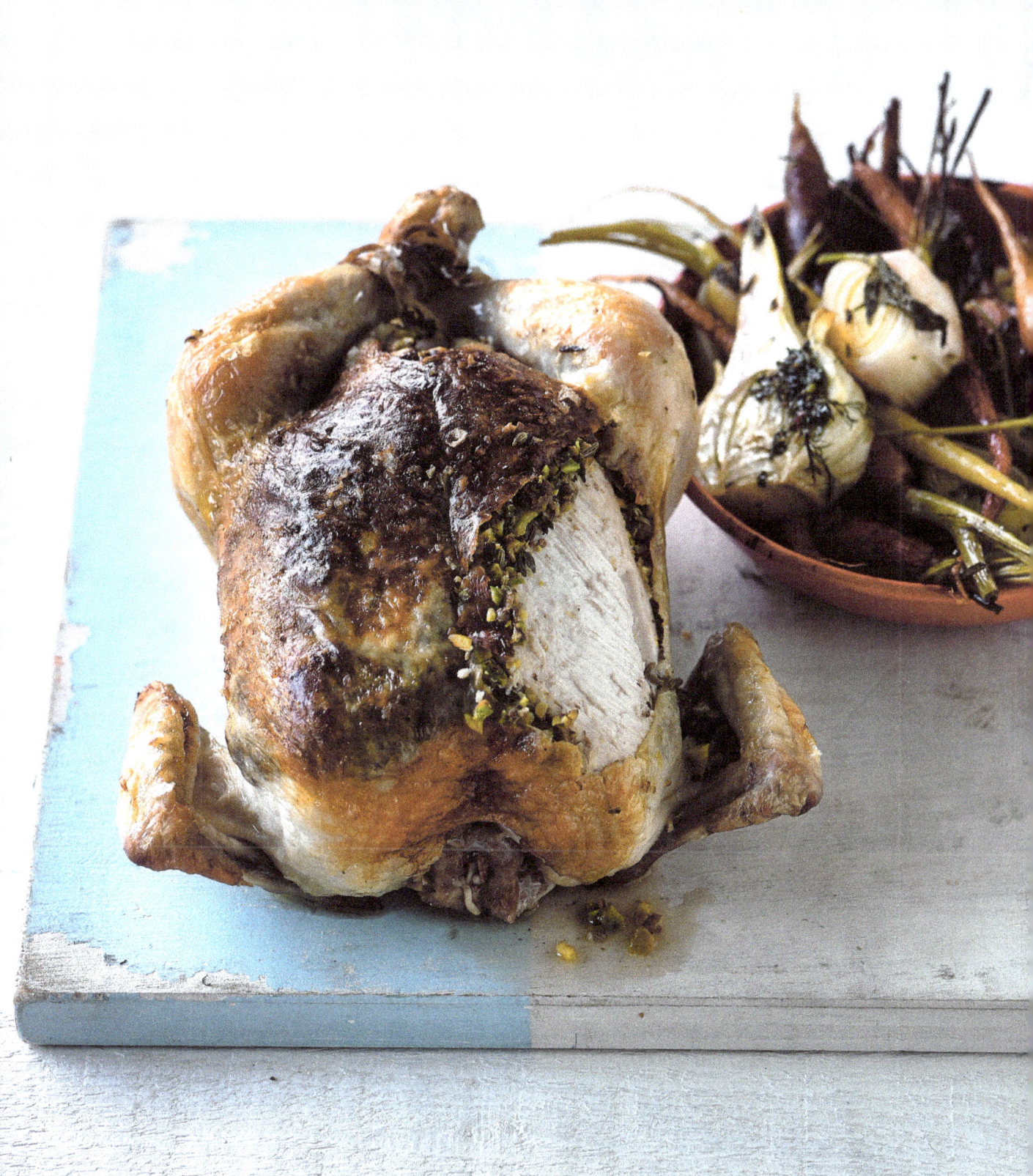

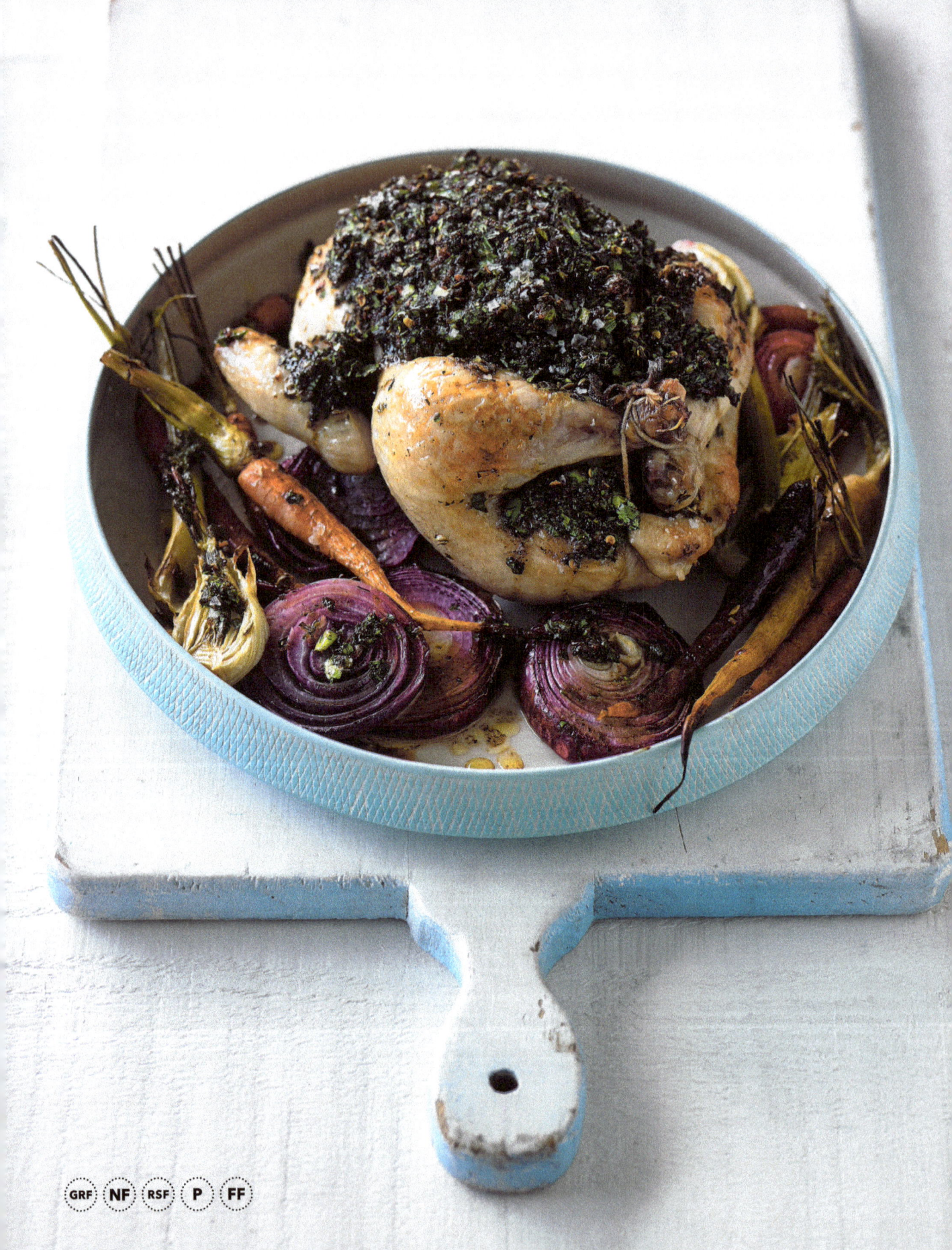

Jerk Chicken

Time to prepare: 30 minutes
Time to cook: 1 hour + 15 minutes to rest

1. Preheat your oven for a good 15 minutes to 200°C/180°C fan-forced.
2. Combine your allspice, pepper, chilli, ginger, garlic, syrup, coriander, parsley and green onions together in a bowl. Season with sea salt.
3. Pop your carrot, fennel and red onion into a large heavy-based roasting pan.
4. Using kitchen paper towels, pat dry your chicken inside and out, tie legs together, then rest chicken on top of vegetables in pan. Season with sea salt and freshly ground black pepper.
5. Stir softened butter, fennel seeds and tarragon together, then spread mixture all over the breast area and legs of the chicken. Squeeze the lemon halves all over, then place into chicken cavity. Pour ½ cup of water into base of pan (this will help steam-roast the vegetables for you).
6. Roast chicken for 30 minutes, then spread your allspice mixture all over chicken and roast for 30 minutes more. Remove from oven and insert a skewer into thigh meat to see if the juice runs clear, if it is still tinged pink then return to oven to roast for another 15 minutes before testing again. Your chicken should have lovely crisp golden skin and tender moist meat. Once removed from oven, stand at room temperature lightly covered in foil for 15 minutes to allow the meat to rest. Serve at table and carve as needed, providing a large spoon for scooping up all the delicious vegetables and pan juices.

SERVES: 6

2 teaspoons ground allspice
2 teaspoons ground black pepper
2 teaspoons dried chilli flakes
3cm piece ginger, peeled and finely grated
2 cloves garlic, peeled and crushed
¼ cup 100% maple syrup
½ small bunch fresh coriander, leaves chopped
½ small bunch fresh flat-leaf parsley, leaves chopped
2 green onions, finely chopped
2 bunches mixed baby carrots, trimmed and skins scrubbed
3 baby fennel, trimmed and thickly sliced lengthwise
2 red onions, peeled and sliced into rounds
1.3 kg fresh organic whole chicken
80g butter, at room temperature
2 teaspoons fennel seeds
1 small bunch fresh tarragon, leaves chopped
1 lemon, halved

Steam-roasted Chinese Chicken

Time to prepare: 20 minutes
Time to cook: 1 hour + 15 minutes to rest

1. Preheat your oven for a good 15 minutes to 200°C/180°C fan-forced.
2. Pop your leek, carrot and zucchini into a large heavy-based roasting pan and season with sea salt and freshly ground black pepper.
3. Using kitchen paper towels, pat dry your chicken inside and out, tie legs together, then rest your chicken on top of your vegetables in pan.
4. Brush chicken all over with your sesame oil. Add your tamari and stock to the roasting pan. Cover the chicken with a large piece of non-stick baking paper, then doubled pieces of foil and wrap tightly.
5. Roast your chicken for 1 hour. Remove from oven and insert a skewer into the thigh meat to see if the juice runs clear, if it is still tinged pink then return to the oven to roast for another 15 minutes before testing again. Once removed from the oven add your bok choy to the pan. Return coverings and stand at room temperature for 15 minutes to allow the meat to rest and bok choy to wilt. Serve at the table and carve as needed. Don't forget to provide a large spoon for scooping up all the delicious vegetables and pan juices.

SERVES: 6

2 leeks, trimmed, rinsed and thickly sliced
2 bunches mixed baby carrots, trimmed and skins scrubbed
3 small zucchini, halved lengthwise
1.3 kg fresh organic whole chicken
3 teaspoons sesame oil
¼ cup tamari
2 cups chicken stock (homemade see recipe pg 51 or organic store bought)
1 bunch baby bok choy, leaves separated

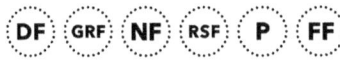

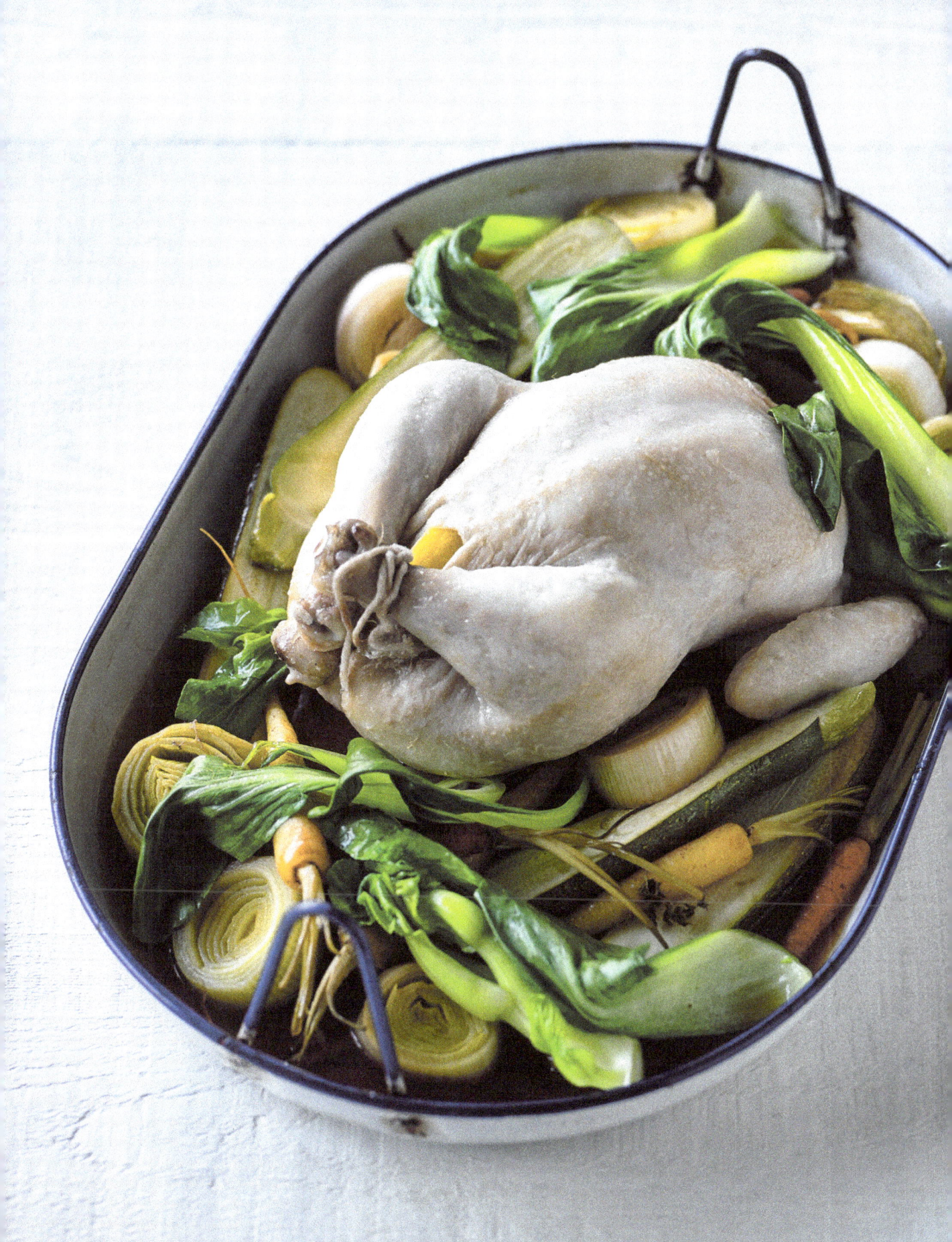

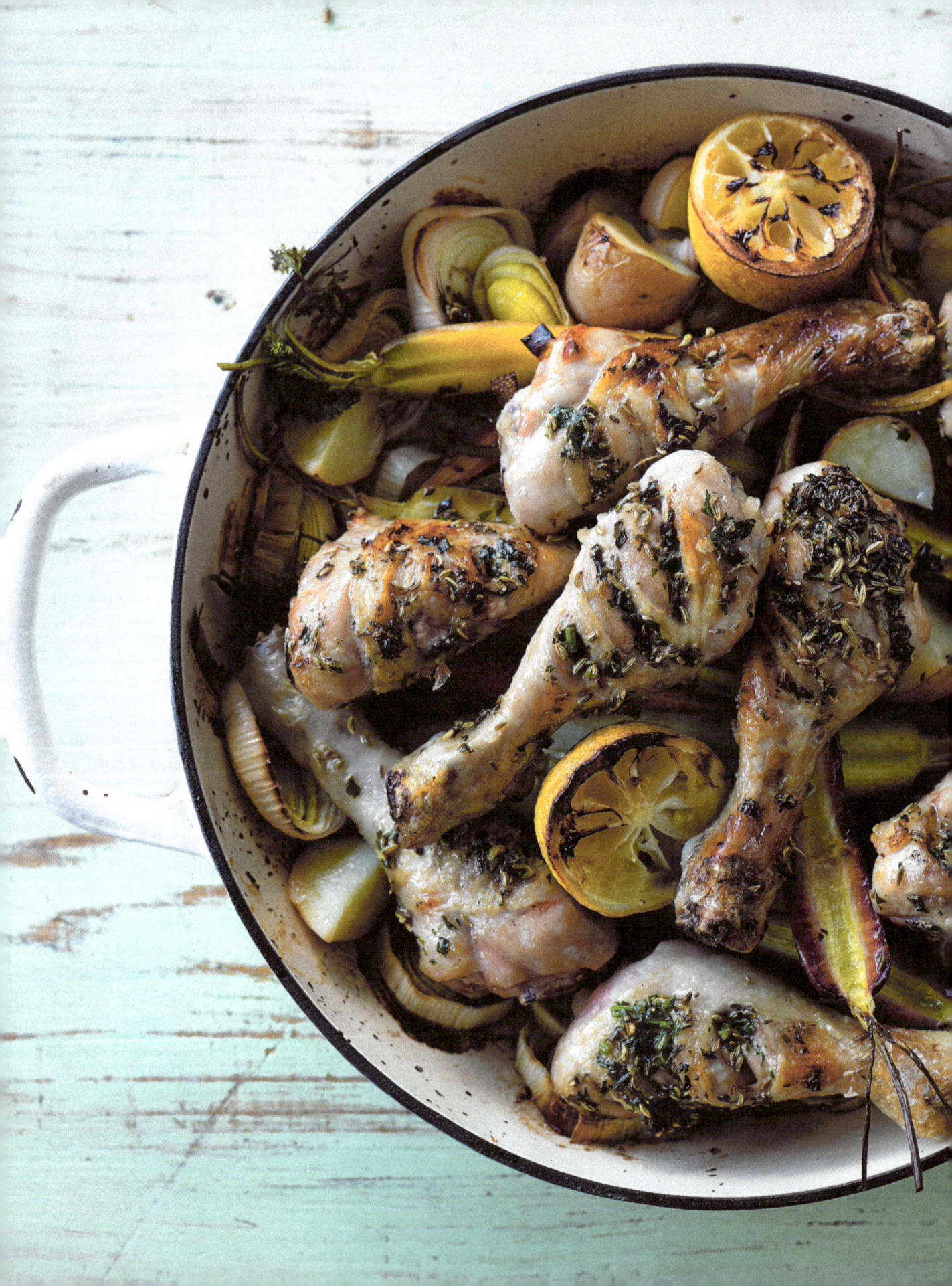

Weeknight Roast Chicken

Time to prepare: 20 minutes
Time to cook: 40 minutes + 10 minutes to rest

1. Preheat your oven for a good 15 minutes to 200°C/180°C fan-forced.
2. Pop your leek, carrot and potato into a large heavy-based roasting pan. Season with sea salt and freshly ground black pepper.
3. Rest your chicken on top of your vegetables in pan. Season with sea salt and freshly ground black pepper.
4. Stir the softened butter, fennel seeds and tarragon together, then spread the mixture all over the drumsticks. Squeeze the lemon halves all over, then place into pan with the vegetables. Pour ½ cup of water into the base of the pan (this will help to steam roast the vegetables for you).
5. Roast your chicken for 40 minutes, turning occasionally, or until cooked and golden. Your chicken should have a lovely crisp golden skin and tender moist meat. Once removed from oven, stand at room temperature, lightly covered with foil, for 10 minutes to allow the meat to rest. Serve the pan straight to the table, providing a large spoon for scooping up all the delicious vegetables and pan juices.

SERVES: 6

2 leeks, trimmed, rinsed and thinly sliced
2 bunches mixed baby carrots, trimmed, skins scrubbed and halved lengthwise
500g baby red potatoes, quartered
8 chicken drumsticks, scored
80g butter, at room temperature
2 teaspoons fennel seeds
1 small bunch fresh tarragon, leaves picked and chopped
1 lemon, halved

(GRF) (NF)   (RSF) (FF)

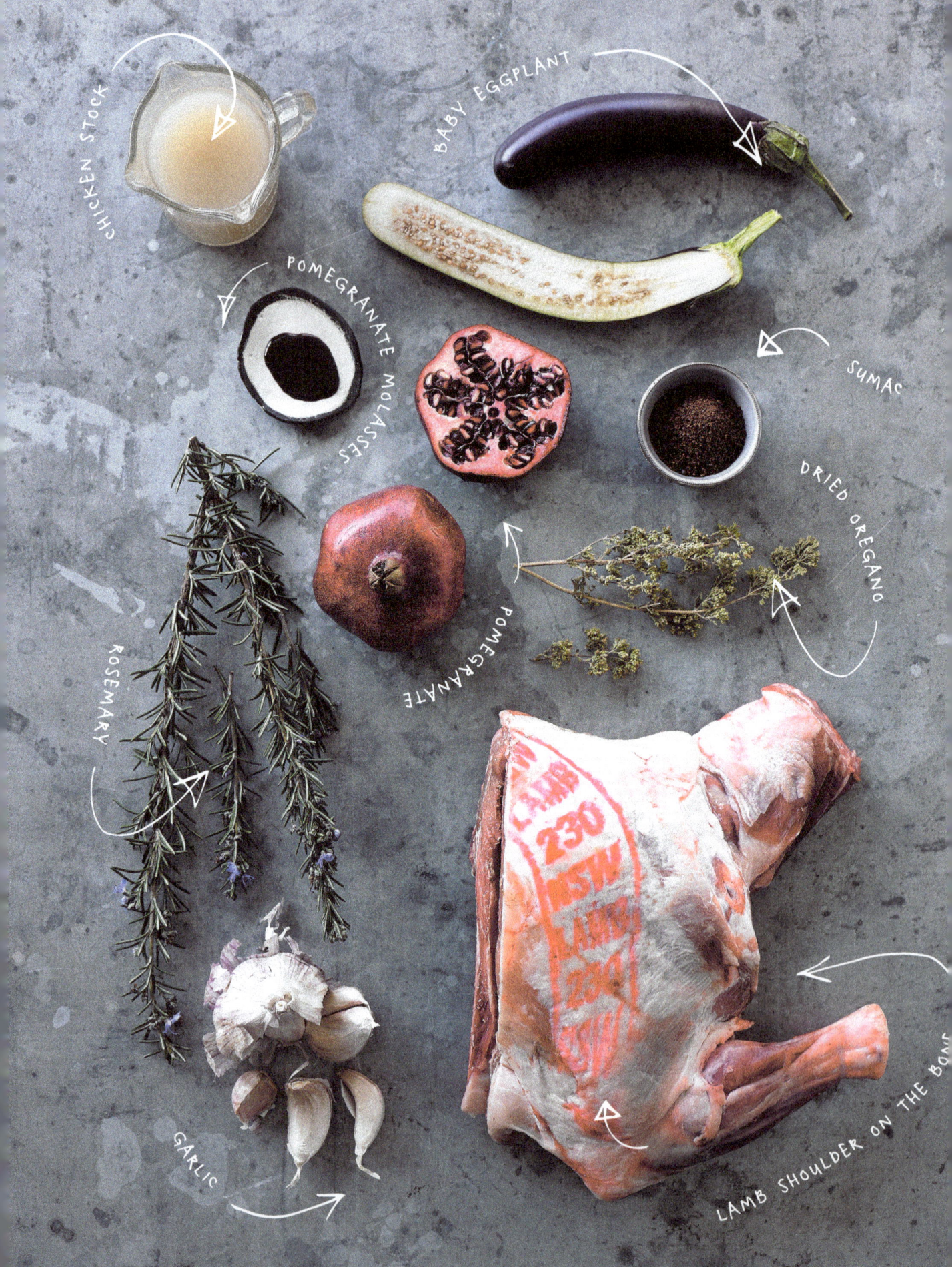

slow-cooking lamb

Basic Slow-cooked Lamb / *66*
Lemony Greek Lamb / *69*
Lamb Salad / *70*
Sumac Lamb / *73*
Make it a Slow-cooker Meal / *74*

ALL ABOUT SLOW-COOKING LAMB

A slow-cooked lamb roast was always the feature of our Sunday dinners growing up and I have kept the same tradition alive with my own family, simply tweaking slightly the different flavour combinations I use. I love the simplicity of the flavours and ease of these recipes. Once again, you simply pop everything in together and slow-roast for 4 hours, without having to do a thing until it is ready to be removed from the oven. Always producing a delicious meal that everyone devours with no mess, no fuss! The perfect end to a week in my mind.

♥ Cuts of lamb you can use

I always use a bone-in cut of lamb such as shoulder or leg when slow-roasting as I find the flavour is always so much nicer when meat is slow-cooked on the bone. However, if you prefer a less messy option when it comes to carving then you can use a boned shoulder or easy carve leg. Just check these cuts after 3 hours of cooking as they tend to cook quicker without the bone-in.

♥ If you're not a fan of lamb

You can easily swap all of these recipes to either use your favourite cut of beef (topside, bolar blade, brisket) or pork (shoulder or loin).

♥ Want a golden brown crispy top

The problem with slow-cooked meats is that they never have a lovely crispy top to them once all their coverings have been removed after cooking. Easily fixed though. Once your lamb is tender, simply turn up your oven temperature to 220°C/200°C fan-forced, return the lamb and cook, uncovered, for 15 minutes or until golden and crispy.

TRY THIS ...

♥ For an easy large gathering

You can easily double or triple these recipes. If we have lunch guests I like to place the lamb into the oven just before going to bed (around 11pm, and I slow-cook at 120°C/100°C fan-forced for 12 hours, perfect timing for a lunchtime gathering. This also leaves me the morning to organise all the side dishes and set the table, plus the smell in the house throughout the morning as the meat is cooking is literally to die for.

♥ Herbs and lamb

Because lamb has such a wonderful rich flavour it is well suited to being paired with other strong tasting herbs such as thyme, lemon thyme, oregano and marjoram. So why not add some of these along with your rosemary when making these recipes.

Basic Slow-cooked Lamb

Time to prepare: 15 minutes
Time to cook: 4 hours + 15 minutes to rest

1. Preheat your oven for a good 15 minutes to 150°C/130°C fan-forced.

2. Pop your celery, onion, carrot, parsley and garlic into a large heavy-based roasting pan. Season with sea salt and freshly ground black pepper. Rest your lamb on top of your vegetables in the pan and sprinkle with your rosemary. Season with sea salt and freshly ground black pepper. Pour your stock into the base of the pan. Cover the lamb with a large piece of non-stick baking paper, then doubled pieces of foil and wrap tightly.

3. Slow-cook your lamb for 4 hours. Remove from oven and if the meat easily falls apart when tested with two forks it's ready. If the meat still feels tight then return to the oven for another 30 minutes before testing again. Once removed from the oven, stand at room temperature, covered, for 15 minutes to allow the meat to rest. Serve at the table and pull apart as needed, providing a large spoon for scooping up all the delicious vegetables and pan juices.

SERVES: 6

3 stalks celery, trimmed, washed and cut into 5cm lengths
2 red onions, peeled and cut into thick wedges
2 carrots, trimmed, roughly cut into 5cm pieces
1 small bunch flat-leaf parsley, stems and leaves chopped
10 cloves garlic, peeled
2kg lamb shoulder on the bone
½ small bunch rosemary, leaves picked
1 cup chicken stock (homemade see recipe pg 51 or store bought organic)

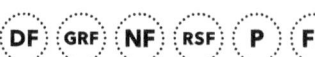

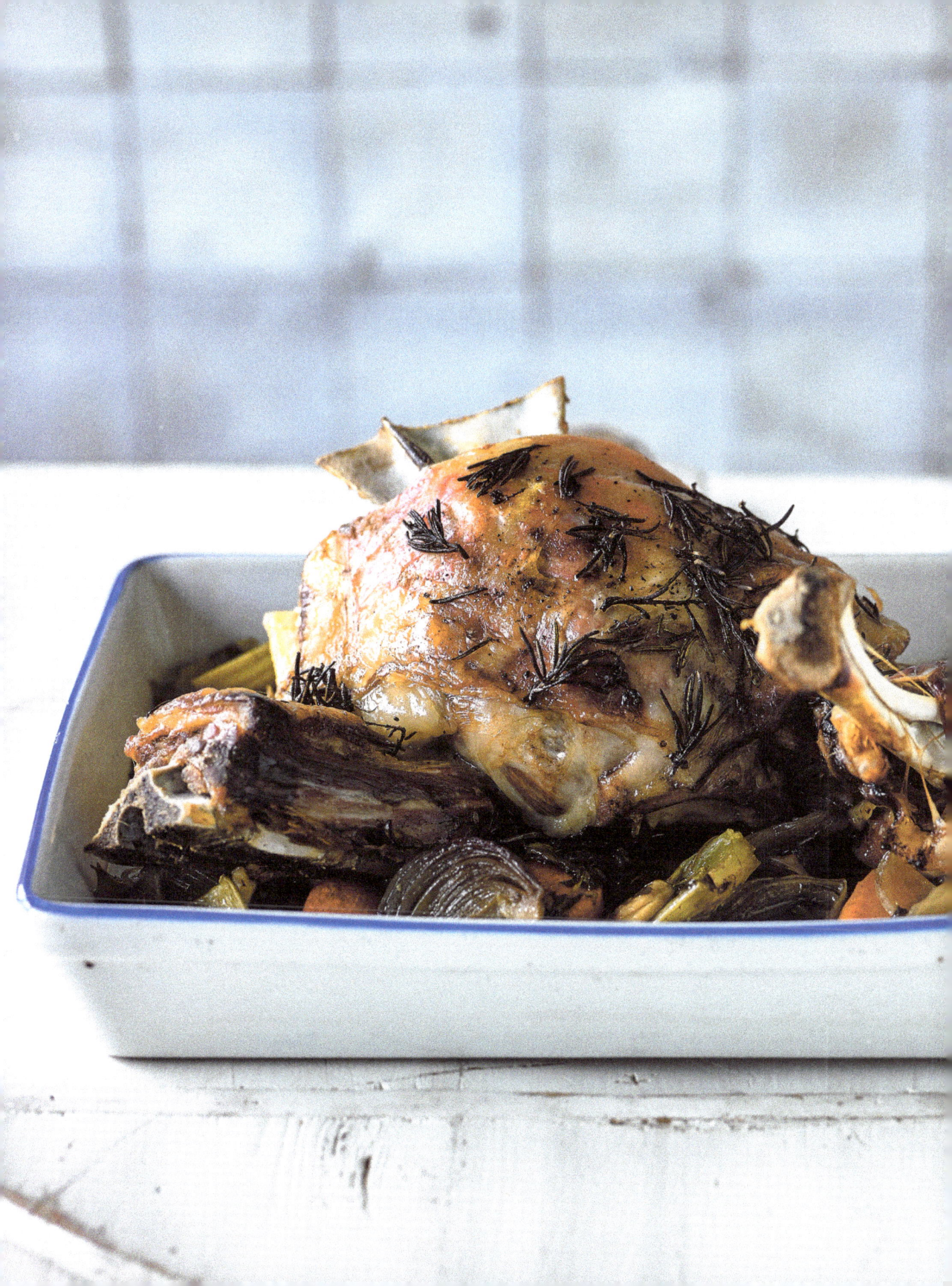

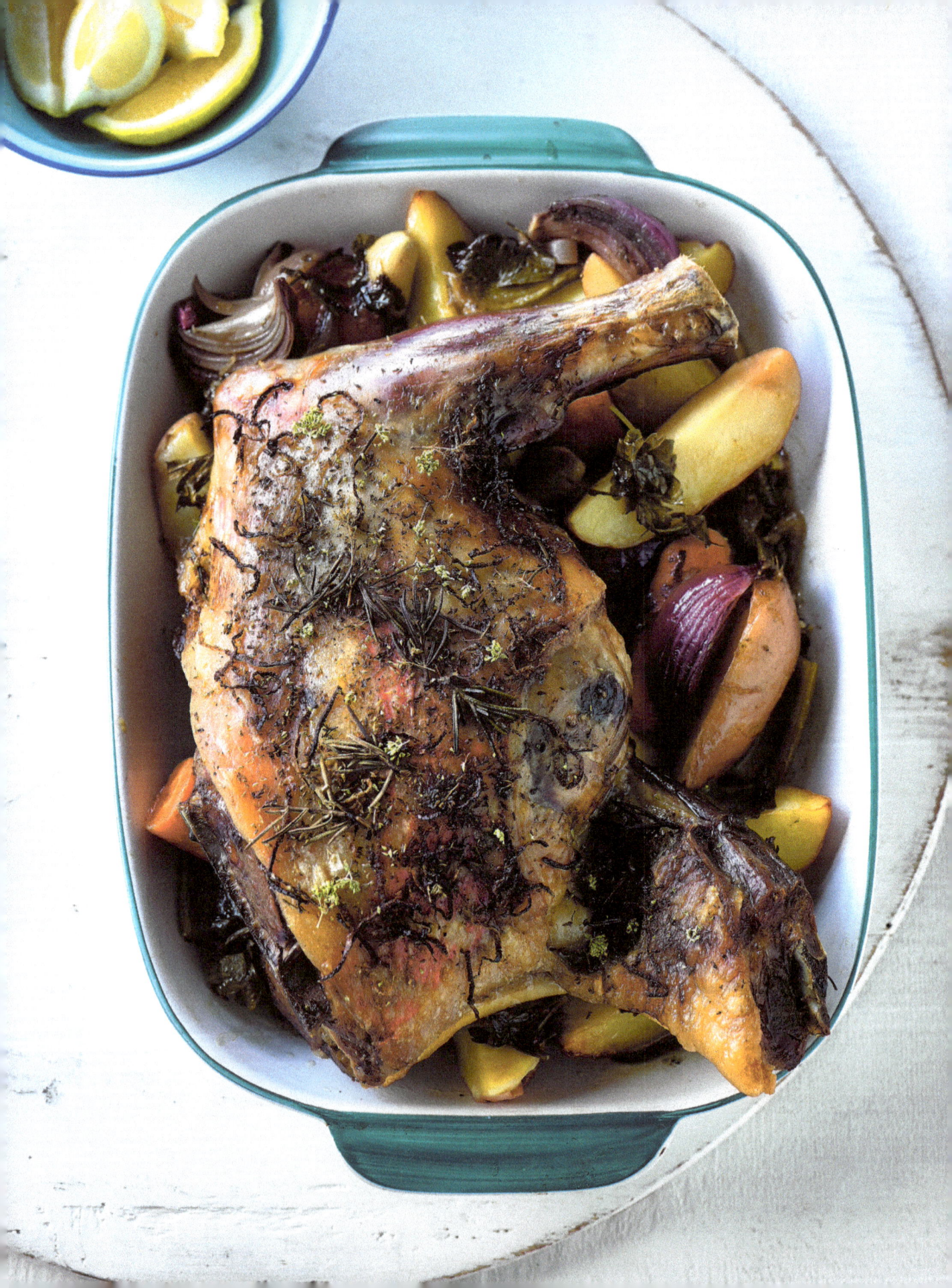

Lemony Greek Lamb

Time to prepare: 20 minutes
Time to cook: 4 hours + 15 minutes to rest

1. Preheat your oven for a good 15 minutes to 150°C/130°C fan-forced.

2. Pop your celery, onion, carrot, parsley and garlic into a large heavy-based roasting pan. Season with sea salt and freshly ground black pepper. Rest your lamb on top of your vegetables in the pan and sprinkle with your rosemary, oregano, lemon zest and juice. Season with sea salt and freshly ground black pepper. Pour your stock into the base of the pan. Cover the lamb with a large piece of non-stick baking paper, then doubled pieces of foil and wrap tightly.

3. Slow-cook your lamb for 3 hours, then add your potato to the pan. Cook for another 1 hour. Remove from oven and if the meat easily falls apart when tested with two forks it's ready. If the meat still feels tight then return to the oven for another 30 minutes before testing again. Once removed from the oven, stand at room temperature, covered, for 15 minutes to allow the meat to rest. Serve at the table sprinkled with your extra oregano, lemon wedges alongside and pull apart as needed, providing a large spoon for scooping up all the delicious vegetables and pan juices.

SERVES: 6

3 stalks celery, trimmed, washed and cut into 5cm lengths
2 red onions, peeled and cut into thick wedges
2 carrots, trimmed, roughly cut into 5cm pieces
1 small bunch flat-leaf parsley, stems and leaves chopped
10 cloves garlic, peeled
2kg lamb shoulder on the bone
½ small bunch fresh rosemary, leaves picked
3 teaspoons dried oregano, plus 1 teaspoon extra
2 lemons, peel zested into strips and juiced
1 cup chicken stock (homemade see recipe pg 51 or store bought organic)
3 large desiree potatoes, quartered lengthwise
Lemon wedges, to serve

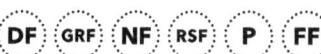

Lamb Salad

Time to prepare: 20 minutes
Time to cook: 4 hours + 15 minutes to rest

1. Preheat your oven for a good 15 minutes to 150°C/130°C fan-forced.
2. Pop celery, onion, carrot, parsley and garlic into a large heavy-based roasting pan. Season with sea salt and freshly ground black pepper. Rest your lamb on top of vegetables in the pan and sprinkle with rosemary and sweet paprika. Season with salt and freshly ground black pepper. Pour stock into the base of the pan. Cover the lamb with a large piece of non-stick baking paper, then doubled pieces of foil and wrap tightly.
3. Slow-cook lamb for 3 hours, then add your eggplant and capsicum to the pan. Cook for another 1 hour. Remove from oven and if the meat easily falls apart when tested with two forks it's ready. If the meat still feels tight then return to the oven for another 30 minutes before testing again. Once removed from the oven, stand at room temperature, uncovered, for 30 minutes to allow the meat to rest and cool slightly.
4. Pull the meat off the bone and thickly shred, discarding bone. Toss all of the meat with the vegetables and pan juices. Transfer to a serving platter and top with the kale leaves and olives. Serve at the table.

SERVES: 6

3 stalks celery, trimmed, washed and cut into 5cm lengths
2 red onions, peeled and cut into thick wedges
2 carrots, trimmed, roughly cut into 5cm pieces
1 small bunch flat-leaf parsley, stems and leaves chopped
10 cloves garlic, peeled
2kg lamb shoulder on the bone
½ small bunch fresh rosemary, leaves picked
3 teaspoons sweet paprika
1 cup chicken stock (homemade see recipe pg 51 or store bought organic)
3 baby eggplant, halved lengthwise
1 red capsicum, seeds removed and thickly sliced
50g baby kale leaves
1 cup un-pitted Sicilian green olives

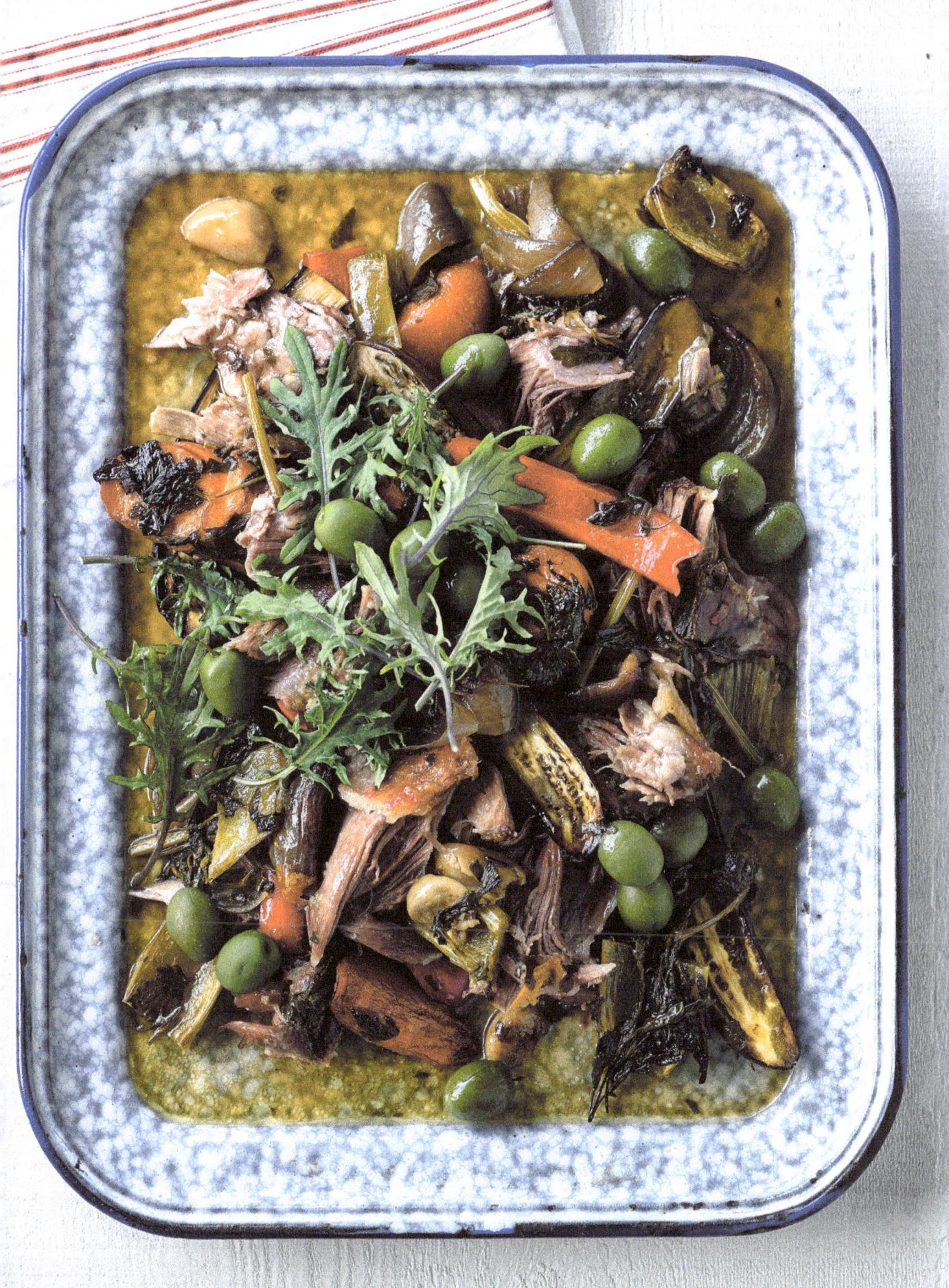

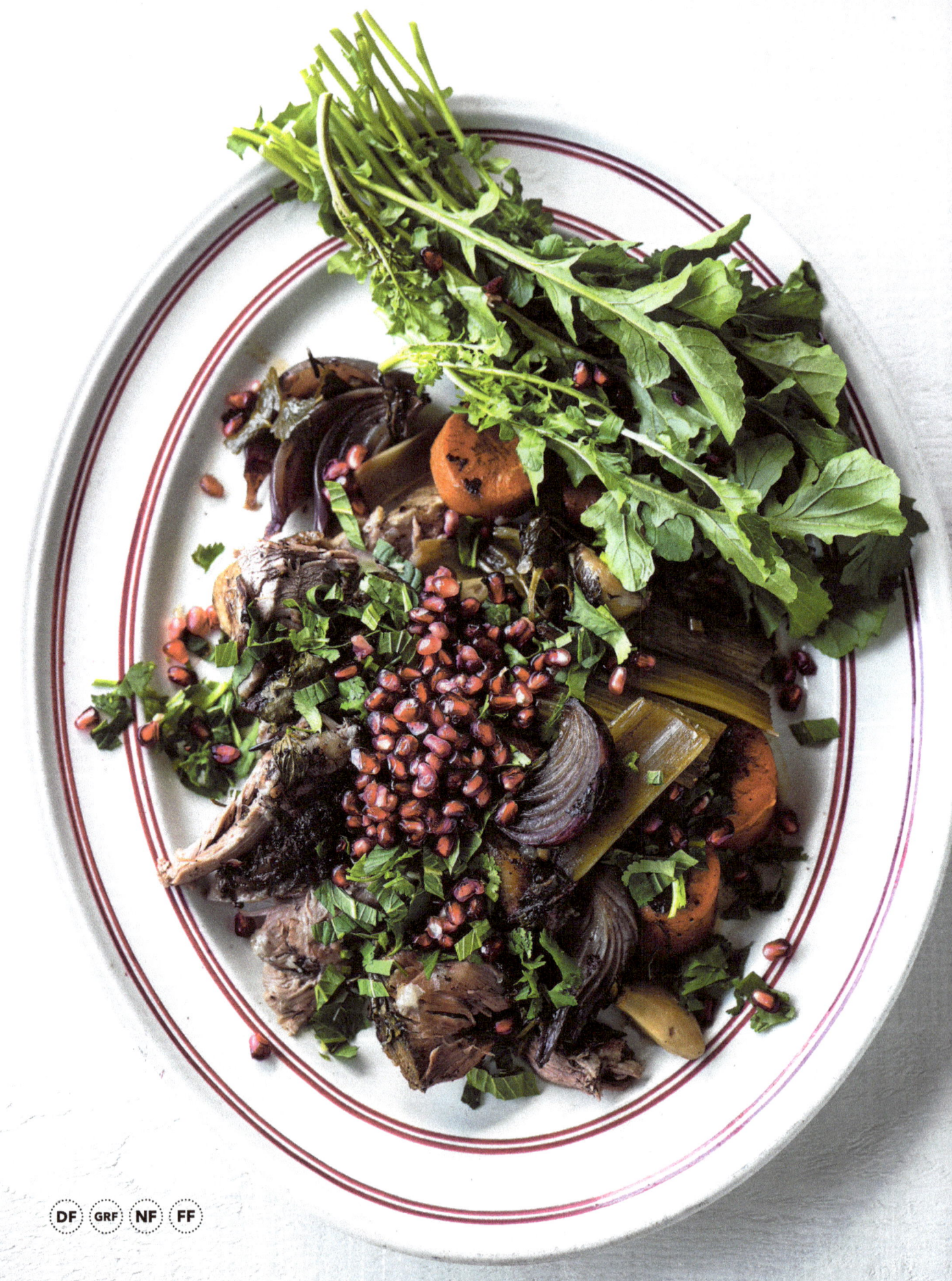

Sumac Lamb

Time to prepare: 25 minutes
Time to cook: 4 hours + 15 minutes to rest

---

1. Preheat your oven for a good 15 minutes to 150°C/130°C fan-forced.

2. Pop your celery, onion, carrot, parsley and garlic into a large heavy-based roasting pan. Season with sea salt and freshly ground black pepper. Rest your lamb on top of your vegetables in the pan and sprinkle with your rosemary, sumac, pomegranate molasses, half of your coriander and half of your mint. Season with salt and freshly ground black pepper. Pour your stock into the base of the pan. Cover the lamb with a large piece of non-stick baking paper, then doubled pieces of foil and wrap tightly.

3. Slow-cook your lamb for 4 hours. Remove from oven and if the meat easily falls apart when tested with two forks it's ready. If the meat still feels tight then return to the oven for another 30 minutes before testing again. Once removed from the oven, stand at room temperature, uncovered, for 15 minutes to allow the meat to rest and cool slightly.

4. Pull the meat off the bone and thickly shred, discarding bone. Toss all of the meat with the vegetables and pan juices. Transfer to a serving platter and sprinkle with your remaining coriander, your remaining mint and your pomegranate seeds. Place your rocket alongside. Serve at the table.

SERVES: 6

3 stalks celery, trimmed, washed and cut into 5cm lengths
2 red onions, peeled and cut into thick wedges
2 carrots, trimmed, roughly cut into 5cm pieces
1 small bunch flat-leaf parsley, stems and leaves chopped
10 cloves garlic, peeled
2kg lamb shoulder on the bone
½ small bunch fresh rosemary, leaves picked
1 tablespoon sumac
2 tablespoons pomegranate molasses
1 small bunch fresh coriander, leaves, stems and roots chopped
1 small bunch fresh mint, leaves picked and chopped
1 cup chicken stock
1 pomegranate, seeds released (see note pg108)
1 bunch rocket, trimmed

HEALTHY MEALS

Make it a Slow-cooker Meal

Time to prepare: 20 minutes + 20 minutes to stand
Time to cook: 4 hours 12 minutes

1. Preheat your slow-cooker for a good 20 minutes on high.
2. Meanwhile, place your beans in a heatproof bowl and pour over enough boiling water to cover, allow to stand for 20 minutes, then drain and rinse under cold running water. Transfer your beans to the slow-cooker.
3. Heat a large deep non-stick frying pan over a high heat. Cook your lamb in 3 separate batches for 2 minutes each or until browned all over. You really want to get a good colour all over the lamb as this adds more flavour and colour to your dish. Transfer your browned lamb to the slow cooker.
4. Reheat the same pan over medium heat. Add your butter, celery, onion, carrot, garlic and rosemary and cook, stirring occasionally, for 5 minutes or until starting to soften. Stir in your stock and remove the pan from the heat. Transfer the vegetable mixture to your slow-cooker, making sure to scrape the bottom of the pan to release all those lovely lamb flavourings.
5. Slow-cook on high, covered, for 4 hours or until the meat is easily falling apart when tested with two forks. Stir through your parsley stems and half of the parsley leaves.
6. Combine the remaining parsley leaves and the extra onion together. Spoon your slow-cooked lamb into a serving dish and sprinkle with your parsley mixture. Serve.

SERVES: 6

1 cup dried black eye beans
600g lamb steaks, cut into 2cm pieces
50g butter
3 stalks celery, trimmed, washed and chopped
1 red onion, peeled and chopped, plus 1 small extra, finely chopped
2 carrots, trimmed, roughly cut into 5cm pieces
10 cloves garlic, peeled
½ small bunch fresh rosemary, leaves picked
2 cups chicken stock (homemade see recipe pg 51 or store bought organic)
1 small bunch flat-leaf parsley, stems and leaves chopped

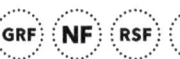

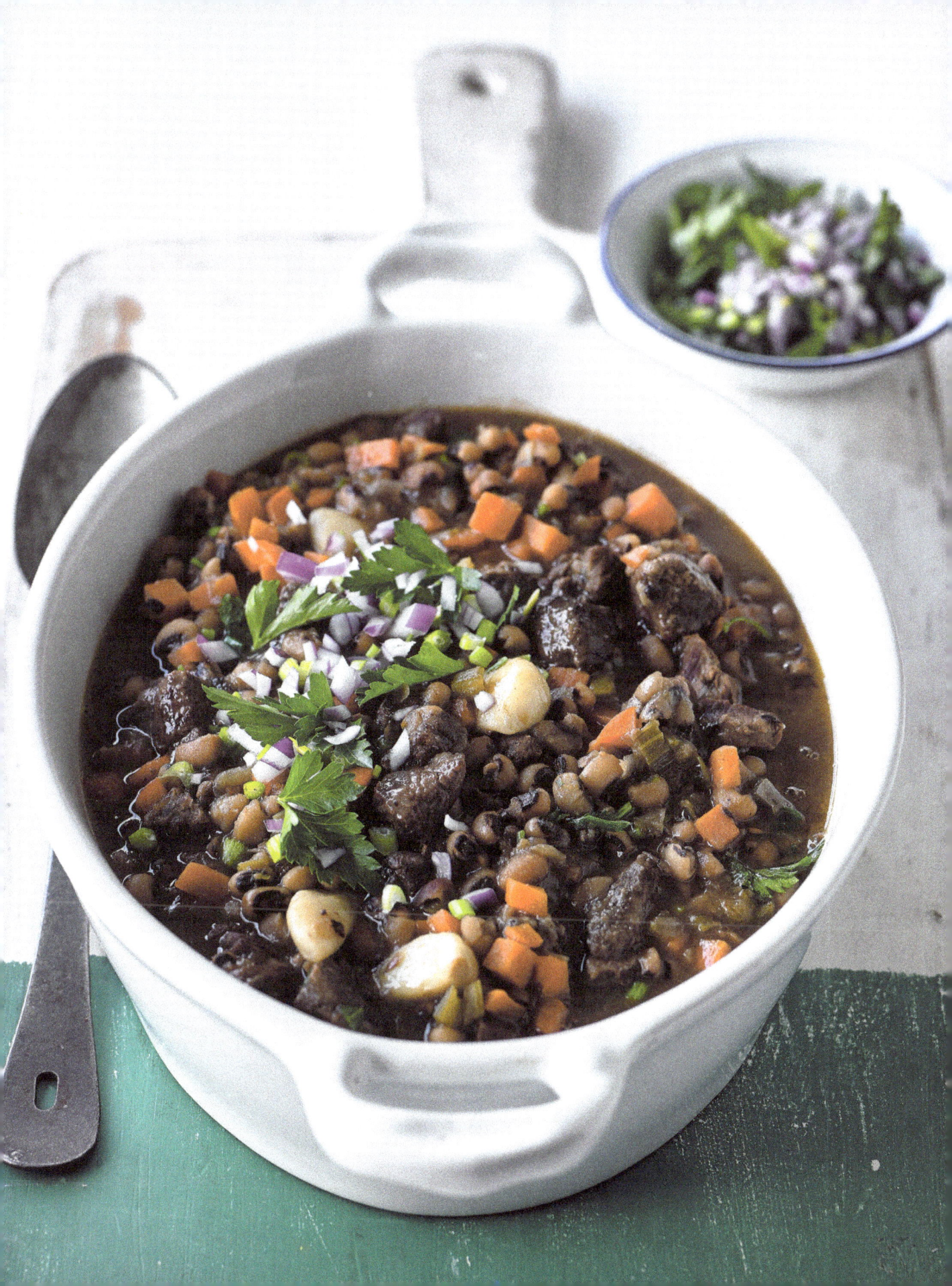

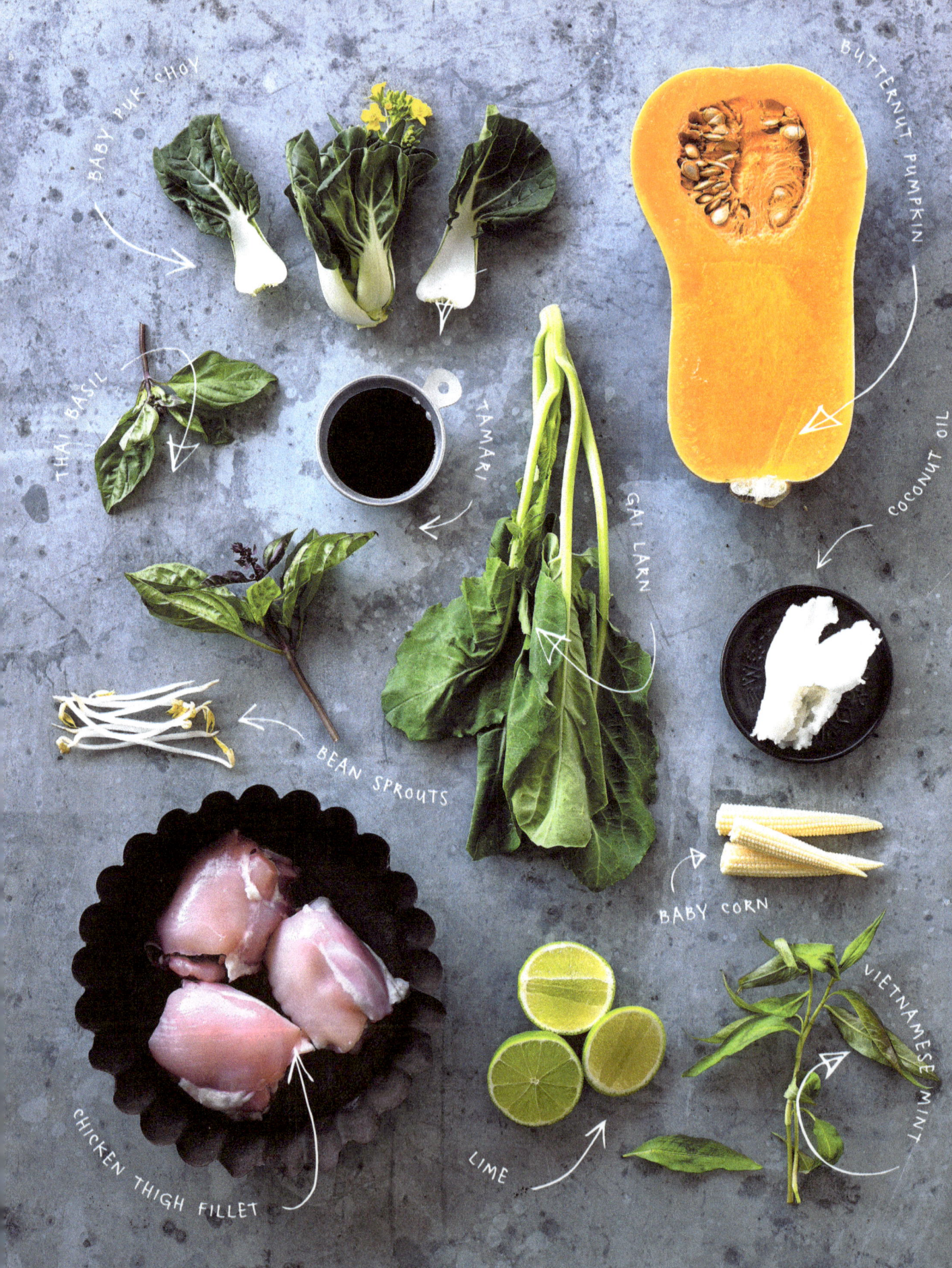

stir-frying chicken

Basic Stir-fry Chicken / *81*

Vietnamese Wraps / *82*

Fried Egg & Stir-fry / *85*

Sweet & Sour Stir-fry / *86*

Stir-fry Salad / *89*

ALL ABOUT STIR-FRYING CHICKEN

I have a confession. I don't own a 'proper' wok to stir-fry in. I use a very large, deep frying pan that has rounded sides which, makes it look like a wok but traditionally not a wok. Once you learn the basics of how to stir-fry and feel confident in cooking them, you literally use whatever cooking vessel you feel most comfortable with. I have used an electric frying pan and a barbecue hotplate to stir-fry in the past when we have been away staying in a cabin.

My top 3 stir-frying tips

- ♥ Have all of your ingredients prepared and ready to go.
- ♥ Get your wok/pan exceptionally hot before you start cooking.
- ♥ Cook your protein in small batches, then allow the wok/pan to get exceptionally hot again between each batch of cooking. This will ensure your meat cooks quickly instead of stewing itself into a grey mass at the base of the wok/pan, keeping it tender to eat.

Why I use chicken thigh fillets

Well they have loads of flavour and the meat never gets dry when you cook them. Plus they have a little fat which helps prevent the meat from sticking to your wok/pan, gets them browning quicker and adds greater flavour to your stir-fry.

Want to stir-fry something other than chicken?

You can either use lamb (fillet, backstrap), pork (fillet, pork leg steaks), beef (rump, fillet), peeled and deveined king prawns or thinly sliced tempeh.

Get more flavour

If you have the time, try marinating your chicken mixture for up to two days in the fridge or freeze for up to 6 months.

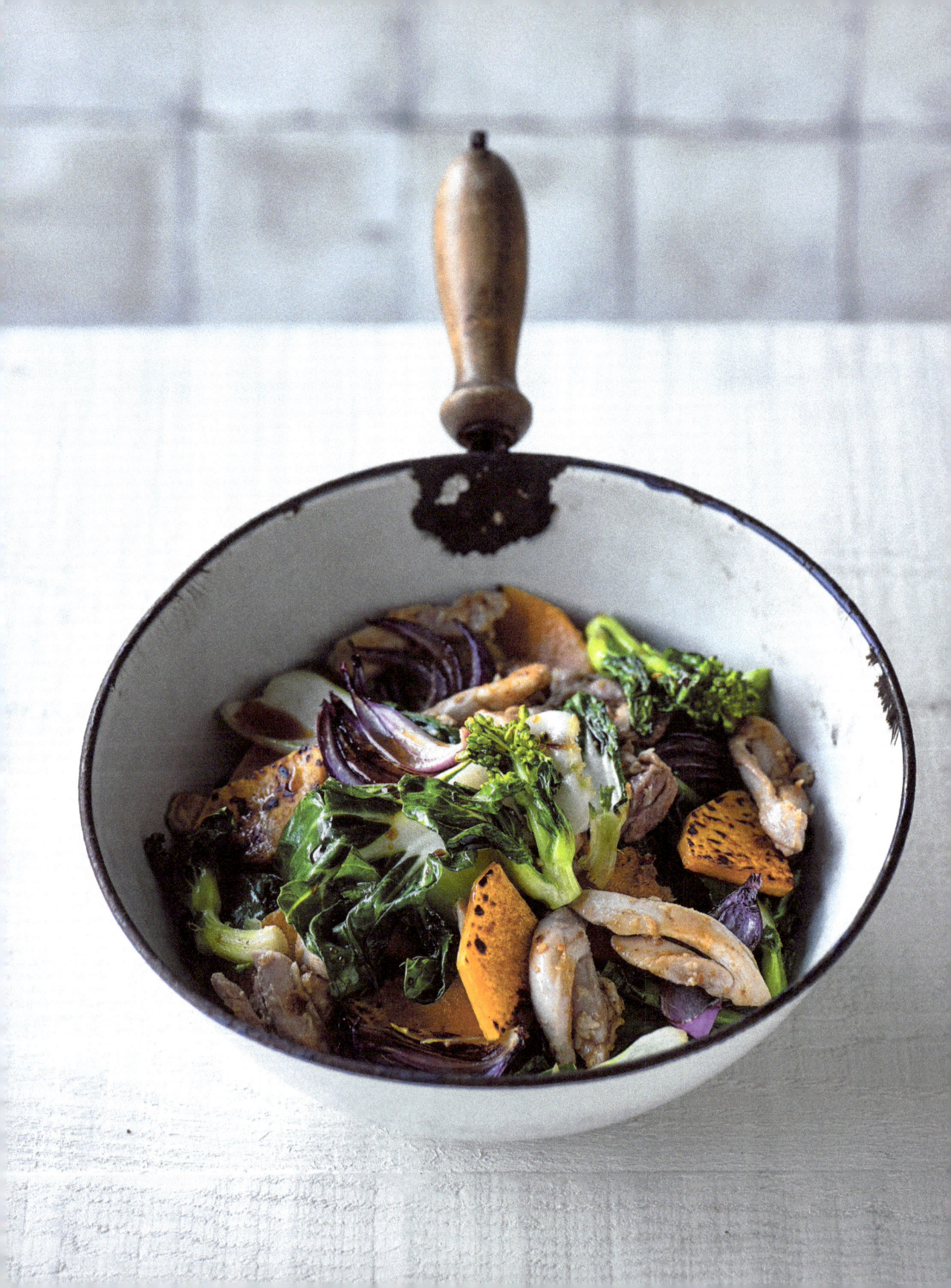

Basic Stir-fry Chicken

Time to prepare 15 minutes + 30 minutes to chill
Time to cook 8 minutes

1. Toss your chicken, garlic, ginger and sesame oil together in a large bowl. Cover the bowl with plastic wrap and chill for 30 minutes to marinate.

2. Preheat your wok over a high heat for a good 3 minutes. Get a second, clean heatproof bowl and place close to your stove top. Add ¼ of your chicken mixture into the very hot wok and using a large heatproof spatula toss around quickly, stir-frying, for 1 minute or until the chicken is almost cooked and starting to colour. Transfer to the clean heatproof bowl. Allow the wok to get extremely hot again, you need to wait 2 minutes for this, then stir-fry another ¼ of your chicken mixture. Repeat this process two more times until all of your chicken has been cooked and is now resting in the heatproof bowl.

3. Re-heat the same wok over a high heat. Add your onion and pumpkin and stir-fry for 2 minutes. Add all your remaining ingredients and stir-fry for 1 minute or until the leaves are just starting to wilt. Return all of your cooked chicken and any of its resting juices to the wok. Stir-fry for another 1 minute to heat through. Serve.

SERVES: 6

500g chicken thigh fillets, thinly sliced crosswise
3 cloves garlic, peeled and crushed
4cm piece fresh ginger, peeled and finely grated
2 teaspoons sesame oil
1 large red onion, peeled and cut into wedges
200g peeled and seeded butternut pumpkin, cut into thin 3cm pieces
1 bunch gai larn, stems cut into 4cm lengths and leaves torn
1 bunch baby puk choy, leaves separated
¼ cup tamari
1 tablespoon honey

(DF) (GRF) (NF) (RSF) (P) (FF)

TRY THESE DELICIOUS IDEAS

Serve your stir-fry with your favourite 'rice' (either cauliflower, brown or white basmati), quinoa, or 'noodles' (zucchini, rice vermicelli or bean thread).

HEALTHY MEALS

Vietnamese Wraps

Time to prepare: 20 minutes + 30 minutes to chill
Time to cook: 7 minutes

1. Toss your chicken, garlic, ginger, sea salt, black pepper, white pepper and sesame oil together in a large bowl. Cover the bowl with plastic wrap and chill for 30 minutes to marinate.

2. Preheat your wok over a high heat for a good 3 minutes. Get a second, clean heatproof bowl and place close to your stove top. Add ¼ of your chicken mixture into the very hot wok and using a large heatproof spatula toss around quickly, stir-frying, for 1 minute or until the chicken is almost cooked and starting to colour. Transfer to the clean heatproof bowl. Allow the wok to get extremely hot again, you need to wait 2 minutes for this, then stir-fry another ¼ of your chicken mixture. Repeat this process two more times until all of your chicken has been cooked and is now resting in the heatproof bowl.

3. Re-heat the same wok over a high heat. Add your onion and pumpkin and stir-fry for 3 minutes or until just starting to soften. Remove your wok from the heat and set aside, allowing the mixture to cool slightly.

4. Arrange your lettuce leaves on a large serving platter and top with your chicken mixture, then bean sprouts and mint. Nestle your lemon wedges in and amongst the filled lettuce leaves, the idea here is that everyone can freshly squeeze their lemons over the top of the wraps just before eating. Serve.

SERVES: 6

500g chicken thigh fillets, cut into 1cm pieces
3 cloves garlic, crushed
4cm piece fresh ginger, peeled and finely grated
2 teaspoons sea salt
2 teaspoons ground black pepper
2 teaspoons ground white pepper
2 teaspoons sesame oil
1 large red onion, peeled, halved and thinly sliced
200g peeled, seeded butternut pumpkin, cut into 1cm pieces
6 iceberg lettuce leaves, trimmed
12 baby cos leaves, trimmed
1½ cups bean sprouts
½ small bunch fresh Vietnamese mint leaves
3 small lemons, cut into 6 wedges

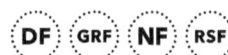

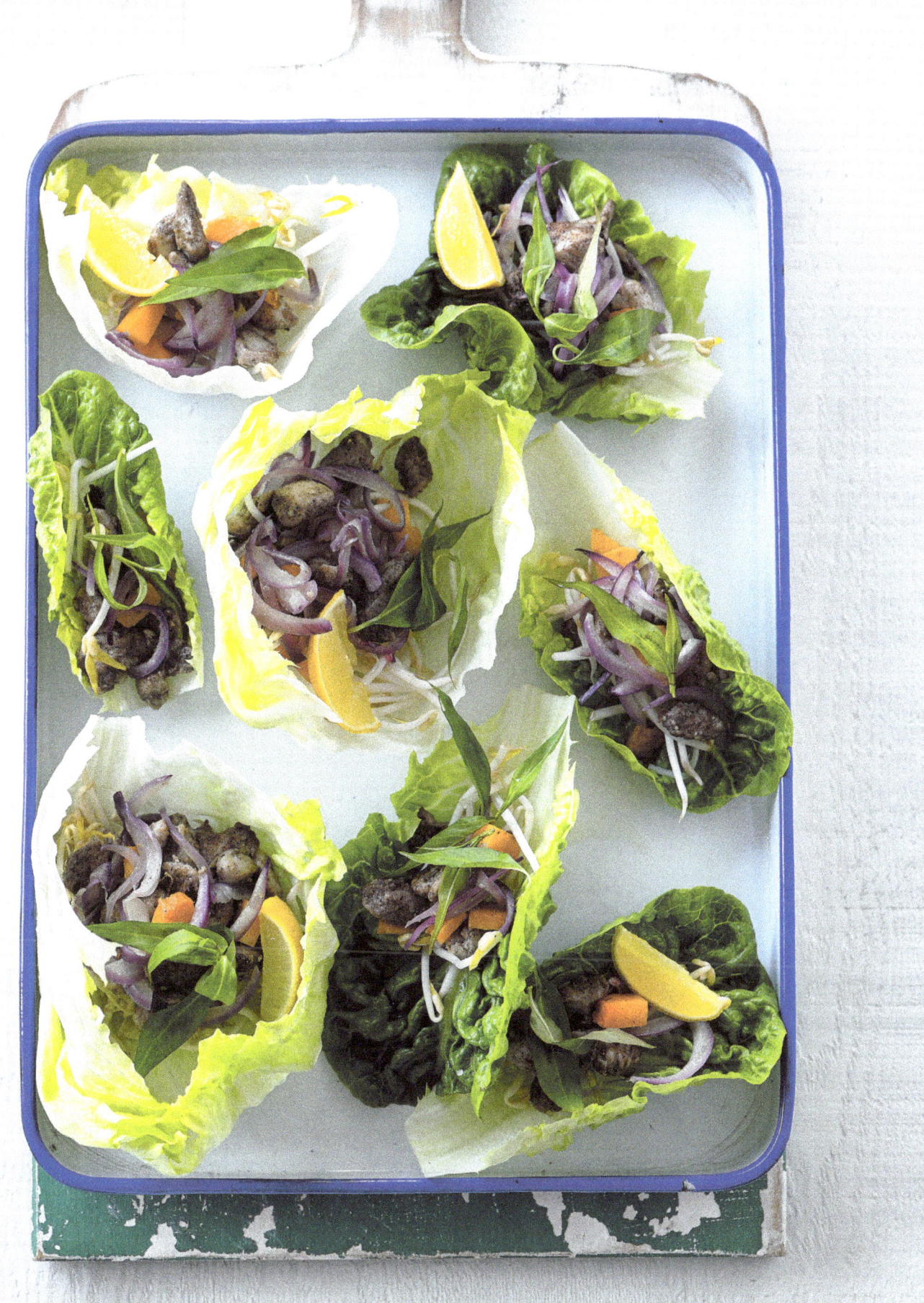

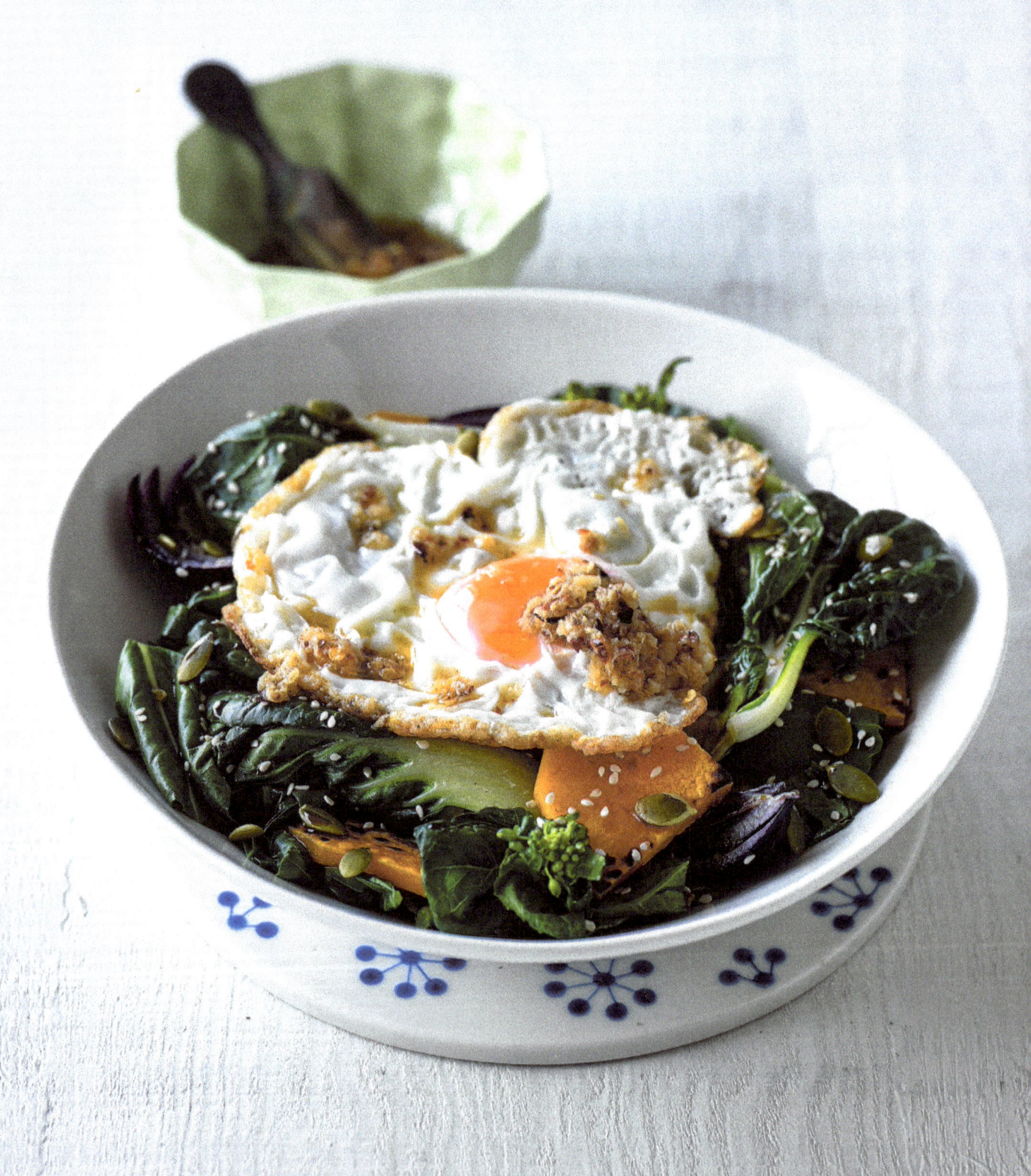

Fried Egg & Stir-fry

Time to prepare: 20 minutes
Time to cook: 11 minutes

1. Combine your garlic, ginger, chilli flakes and sesame oil together in a small bowl. Season with sea salt and freshly ground black pepper. Set aside.

2. Heat a large non-stick frying pan over a medium heat. Add your coconut oil and swirl the pan occasionally until it melts. Crack the eggs into the pan, leaving enough space in between so they don't touch each other and cook, untouched, for 4 minutes or until the egg whites have set and yolks still soft. You can use a spoon to baste the eggwhite with the melted oil in your pan for a super crispy edge. Remove from heat.

3. Preheat your wok over a high heat for a good 3 minutes. Add your onion, pumpkin and ¼ cup water and using a large heatproof spatula toss around quickly, stir-frying, for 3 minutes or until the water has evaporated and the pumpkin is just starting to soften. Add your gai larn, puk choy, tamari and honey and stir-fry for 1 minute or until the leaves are just starting to wilt.

4. Transfer your stir-fried vegetables to serving bowls and sprinkle with your sesame seeds and pepitas. Top with your fried eggs and then drizzle with your sesame oil mixture. Serve.

SERVES: 6

3 cloves garlic, peeled and crushed
4cm piece fresh ginger, peeled and finely grated
1 teaspoon dried chilli flakes
2 tablespoons sesame oil
¼ cup coconut oil
6 eggs
1 large red onion, peeled and cut into wedges
200g peeled and seeded butternut pumpkin, cut into thin 3cm pieces
1 bunch gai larn, stems cut into 4cm lengths and leaves torn
1 bunch baby puk choy, leaves separated
¼ cup tamari
1 tablespoon honey
1 tablespoon sesame seeds
¼ cup pepitas (shelled pumpkin seeds)

HEALTHY MEALS

Sweet & Sour Stir-fry

Time to prepare: 15 minutes + 30 to chill
Time to cook: 7 minutes

1. Toss your chicken, garlic, ginger and sesame oil together in a large bowl. Cover the bowl with plastic wrap and chill for 30 minutes to marinate.

2. Preheat your wok over a high heat for a good 3 minutes. Get a second, clean heatproof bowl and place close to your stove top. Add ¼ of your chicken mixture into the very hot wok and using a large heatproof spatula toss around quickly, stir-frying, for 1 minute or until the chicken is almost cooked and starting to colour. Transfer to the clean heatproof bowl. Allow the wok to get extremely hot again, you need to wait 2 minutes for this, then stir-fry another ¼ of your chicken mixture. Repeat this process two more times until all of your chicken has been cooked and is now resting in the heatproof bowl.

3. Re-heat the same wok over a high heat. Add your onion, capsicum and baby corn and stir-fry for 1 minute. Add all your remaining ingredients and stir-fry for 1 minute or until the leaves are just starting to wilt. Return all of your chicken and any of its resting juices to the wok. Stir-fry for another 1 minute to heat through. Serve.

SERVES: 6

500g chicken thigh fillets, thinly sliced crosswise
3 cloves garlic, peeled and crushed
4cm piece fresh ginger, peeled and finely grated
2 teaspoons sesame oil
1 large red onion, peeled and cut into wedges
1 red capsicum, seeds removed and thinly sliced
125g fresh baby corn, halved lengthwise
1 bunch baby puk choy, leaves separated
1 tablespoon tamari
1 tablespoon honey
1 lime, zest finely grated and juiced

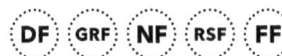

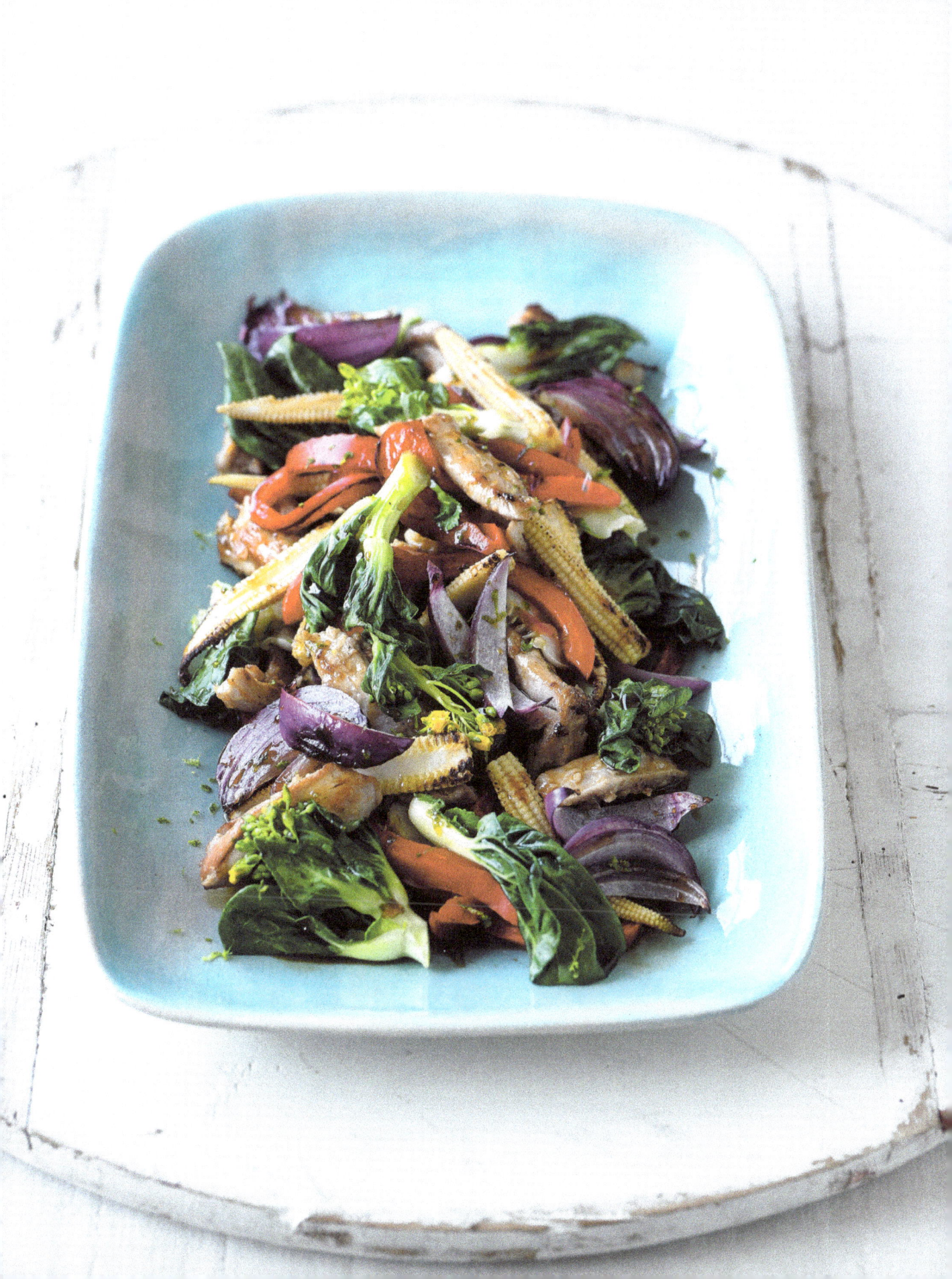

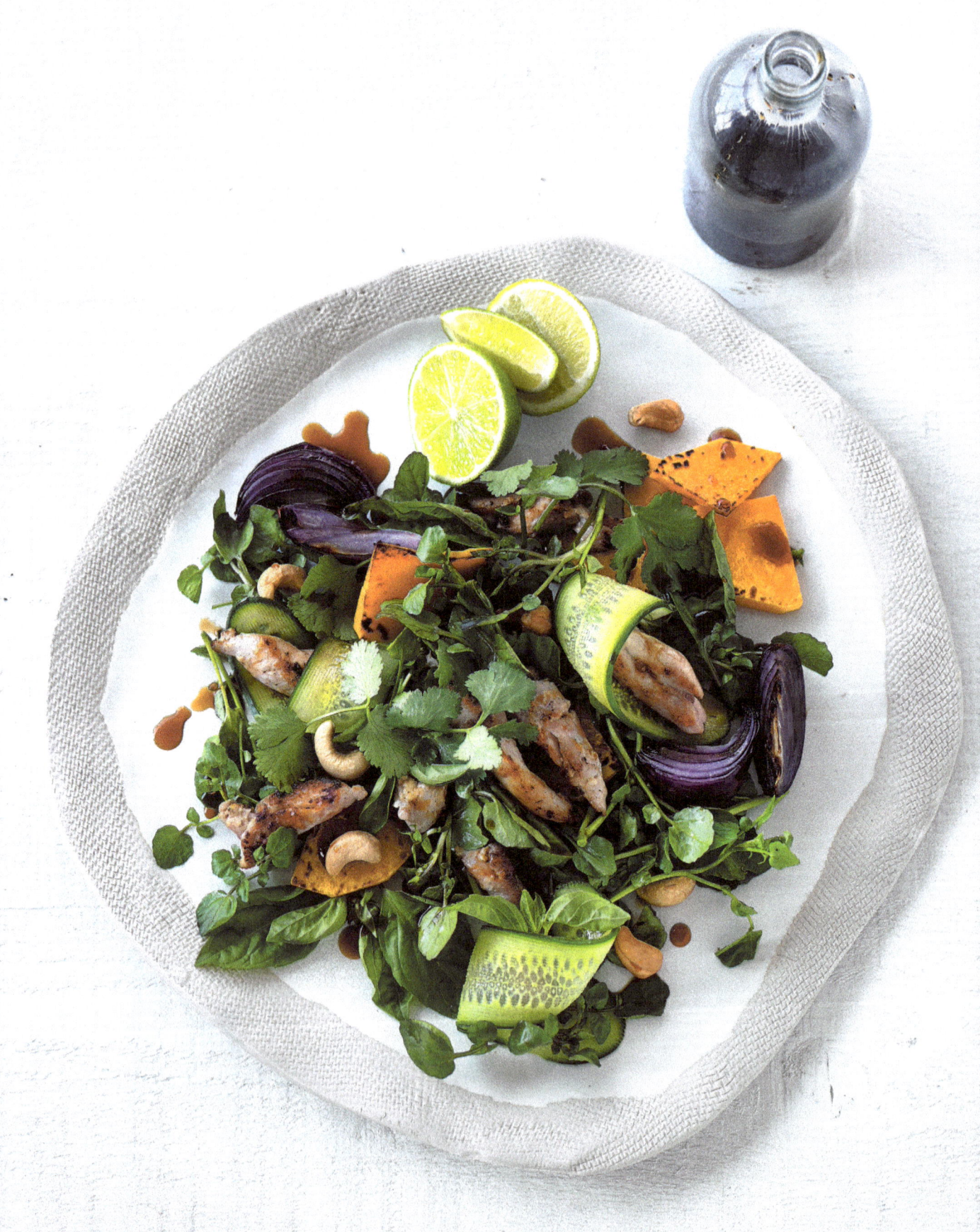

Stir-fry Salad

Time to prepare: 20 minutes + 30 minutes to chill
Time to cook: 6 minutes

SERVES: 6

500g chicken thigh fillets, thinly sliced crosswise
3 cloves garlic, peeled and crushed
4cm piece fresh ginger, peeled and finely grated
2 teaspoons sesame oil
1 large red onion, peeled and cut into wedges
200g peeled and seeded butternut pumpkin, cut into thin 3cm pieces
¼ cup tamari
1 tablespoon honey
1 bunch watercress, trimmed
2 Lebanese cucumbers, peeled into long thin lengths (see note)
1 small bunch fresh coriander, leaves picked
1 small bunch fresh Thai basil, leaves picked
⅓ cup raw cashews, roasted
Lime cheeks, to serve

1. Toss your chicken, garlic, ginger and sesame oil together in a large bowl. Cover the bowl with plastic wrap and chill for 30 minutes to marinate.

2. Preheat your wok over a high heat for a good 3 minutes. Get a second, clean heatproof bowl and place close to your stove top. Add ¼ of your chicken mixture into the very hot wok and using a large heatproof spatula toss around quickly, stir-frying, for 1 minute or until the chicken is almost cooked and starting to colour. Transfer to the clean heatproof bowl. Allow the wok to get extremely hot again, you need to wait 2 minutes for this, then stir-fry another ¼ of your chicken mixture. Repeat this process two more times until all of your chicken has been cooked and is now resting in the heatproof bowl.

3. Re-heat the same wok over a high heat. Add your onion and pumpkin and stir-fry for 1 minute. Add your tamari and honey and stir-fry for 1 minute. Return all of your chicken and any of its resting juices to the wok. Stir-fry until well combined. Remove your wok from the heat and set aside, allowing the mixture to cool slightly.

4. Arrange your watercress, cucumber, coriander, Thai basil and chicken stir-fry mixture onto a serving platter. Serve sprinkled with your cashews and lime cheeks alongside.

RECIPE NOTE Use your vegetable peeler to achieve lovely long thin lengths of cucumber.

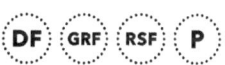

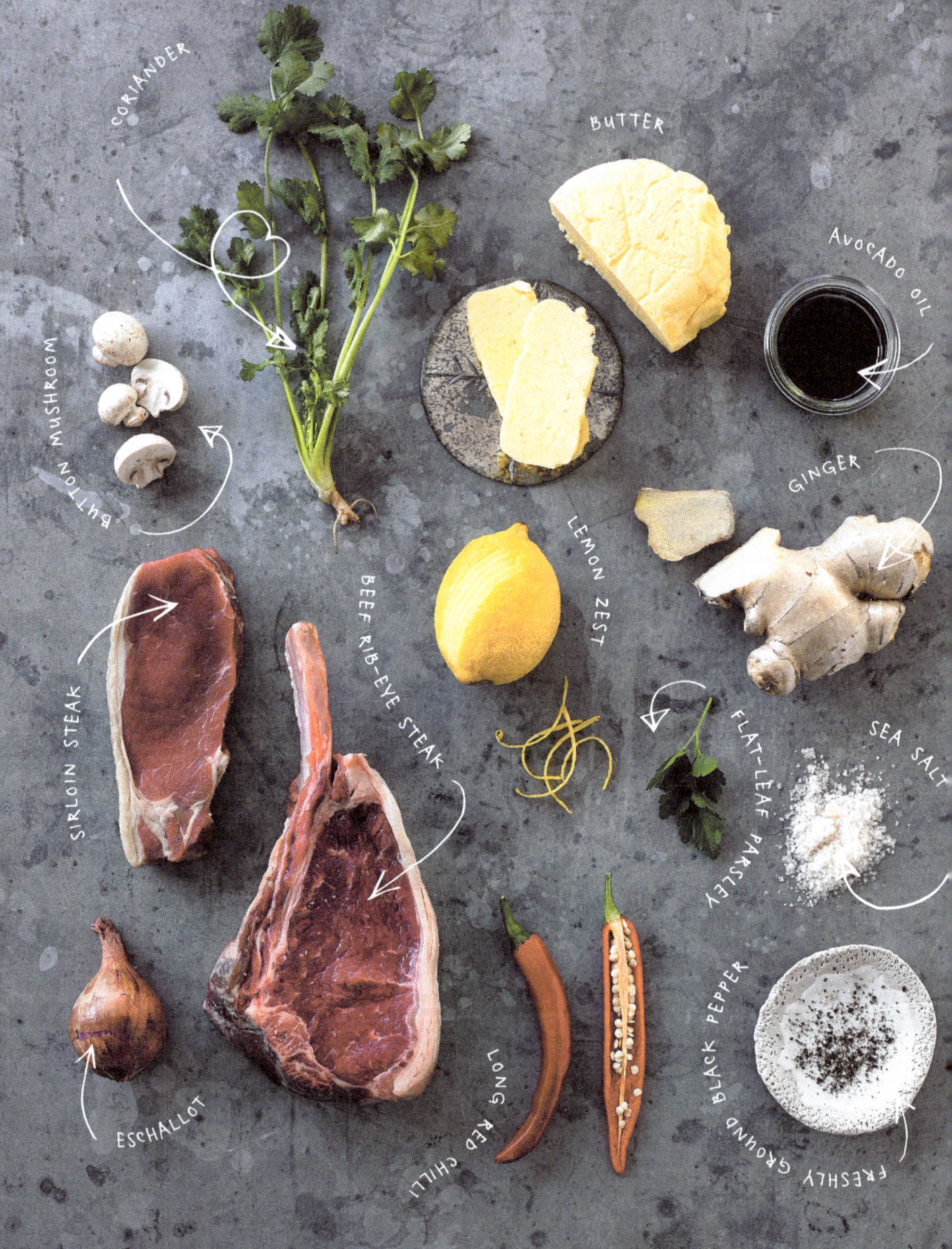

char-grilling steak

Basic Char-grilled Steak / *95*
Gingered Beef / *96*
Adobo Beef / *99*
Beef Bourguignon / *100*
Meat-lovers Rib-eye / *103*

ALL ABOUT CHAR-GRILLING STEAK

Honestly, there is nothing more delicious than a perfectly cooked steak. It's a simple meal that can be enjoyed year round with little effort. Purchase good quality grass-fed beef from your butcher or farmer for maximum flavour. I like to post-marinate my steaks — this means putting them into a marinade mixture once they have been cooked. I allow the steak to sit in the post-marinade while they rest. As the steak rests, the natural juice will then meld with the marinade mixture to form a lovely sauce for drizzling when plated. Just heaven!

My top 3 char-grilling tips

- Always preheat your char-grill pan or barbecue char-grill plate until hot before adding your steak.
- Don't fuss with your meat, allow it to char-grill on one side, turn once, then continue to char-grill on the other side.
- Allow your steak to rest before serving as this allows the meat fibres to relax and reabsorb their juices before serving.

How will I know if it is 'done'

I always find using a timer the best option, but you can also use the tip of your cooking tongs to gently press the flesh too. Rare will feel soft, medium will be springy and a well done steak will feel firm when lightly touched.

Best beef cuts to use for char-grilling

I have used 2cm thick sirloin steaks (also known as porterhouse or New York) in the recipes. You can also use rump, fillet, scotch fillet or t-bone.

Want to char-grill something other than beef?

Always keep the cooking principles the same but adjust your cooking times to suit your new chosen protein. Try Australian sustainable wild caught fish fillets or cutlets (salmon, snapper, and flathead), lamb backstrap or fillet, pork leg steaks or cutlets, tempeh or mixed vegetables (eggplant, capsicum, zucchini, sweet potato).

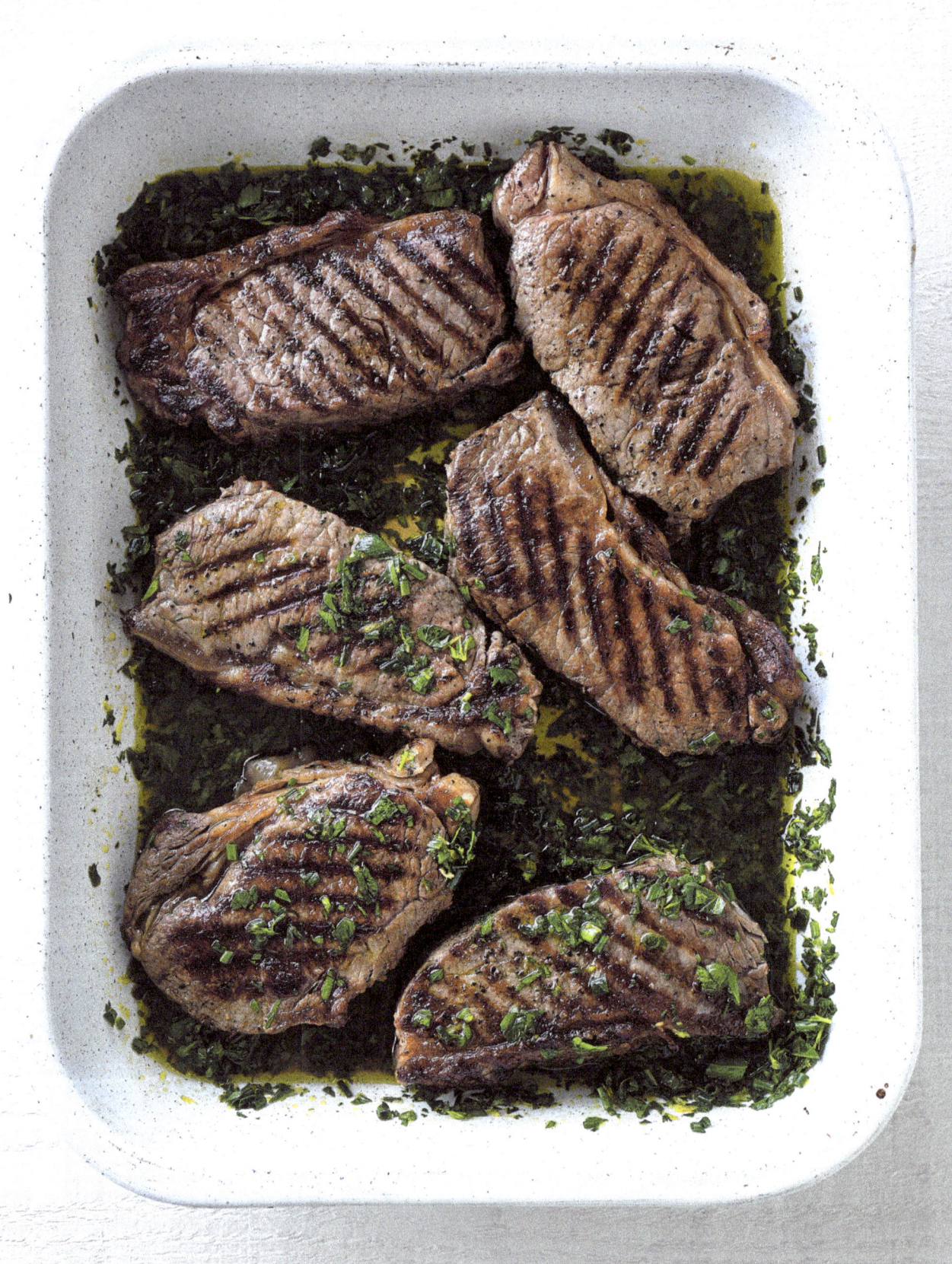

Basic Char-grilled Steak

Time to prepare: 10 minutes
Time to cook: 6 minutes + 6 minutes to rest

1. Season both sides of your steak with sea salt and freshly ground black pepper. Allow to come to room temperature.

2. Pop all of your remaining ingredients together in a glass or ceramic baking dish large enough so that your steaks will fit side by side in a single layer. Season with sea salt and freshly ground black pepper. Set the dressing mixture aside.

3. Preheat a large char-grill pan or barbecue char-grill plate to medium. Once hot, add steaks. Char-grill, untouched (and I mean it here, do not poke or prod steak with tongs, turn or lift slightly to see underneath and do not shuffle it around on your char-grill), for 3 minutes. Turn and char-grill, untouched again, for another 3 minutes for medium-rare.

4. Transfer your steak to the dressing mixture in the dish, making sure they sit side by side in a single layer. Stand for 3 minutes, then gently turn and stand for another 3 minutes until the meat has rested. Serve steak with the lovely dressing mixture spooned over.

SERVES: 6

6 x 300g beef sirloin steaks
½ cup avocado oil
2 large lemons, zest finely grated and then juiced
1 small bunch fresh flat-leaf parsley, leaves finely chopped
1 small bunch fresh chives, thinly sliced

Gingered Beef

Time to prepare: 15 minutes
Time to cook: 6 minutes + 6 minutes to rest

1. Season both sides of your steak with sea salt and freshly ground black pepper. Allow to come to room temperature.

2. Pop all of your remaining ingredients together in a glass or ceramic baking dish large enough so that your steaks will fit side by side in a single layer. Season with sea salt and freshly ground black pepper. Set the dressing mixture aside.

3. Preheat a large char-grill pan or barbecue char-grill plate to medium. Once hot, add your steaks. Char-grill, untouched (and I mean it here, do not poke or prod your steak with tongs, turn or lift slightly to see underneath and do not shuffle it around on your char-grill), for 3 minutes. Turn and char-grill, untouched again, for another 3 minutes for medium-rare.

4. Transfer your steak to the dressing mixture in your dish in a single layer. Stand for 3 minutes, then gently turn and stand for another 3 minutes until the meat has rested. Serve steak with the lovely dressing mixture spooned over.

SERVES: 6

6 x 300g beef sirloin steaks
½ cup avocado oil
2 large lemons, zest finely grated and then juiced
1 small bunch fresh coriander, leaves picked
1 small bunch fresh chives, thinly sliced
5cm piece fresh ginger, peeled and finely grated

(DF) (GRF) (NF) (RSF) (P) (FF)

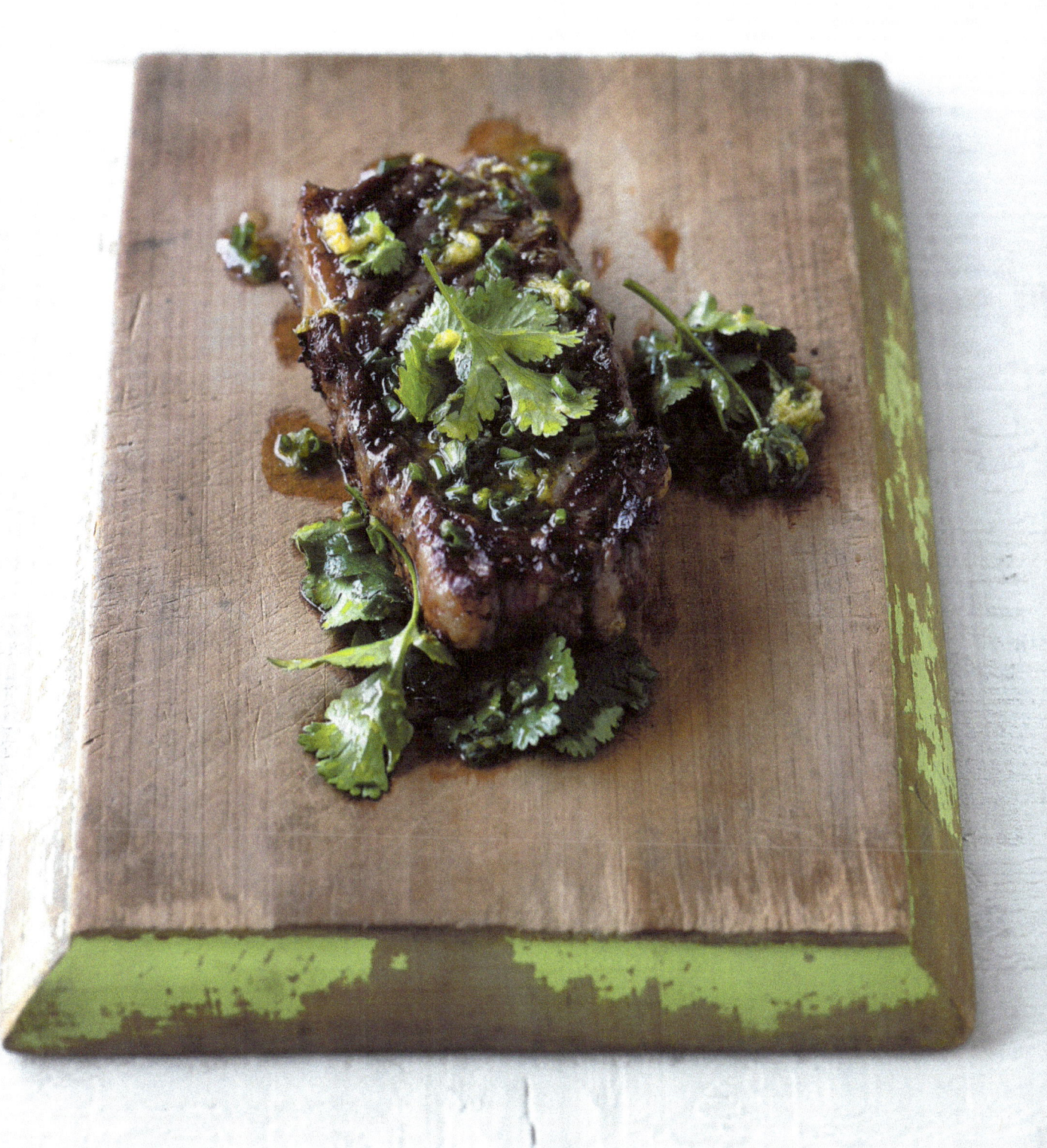

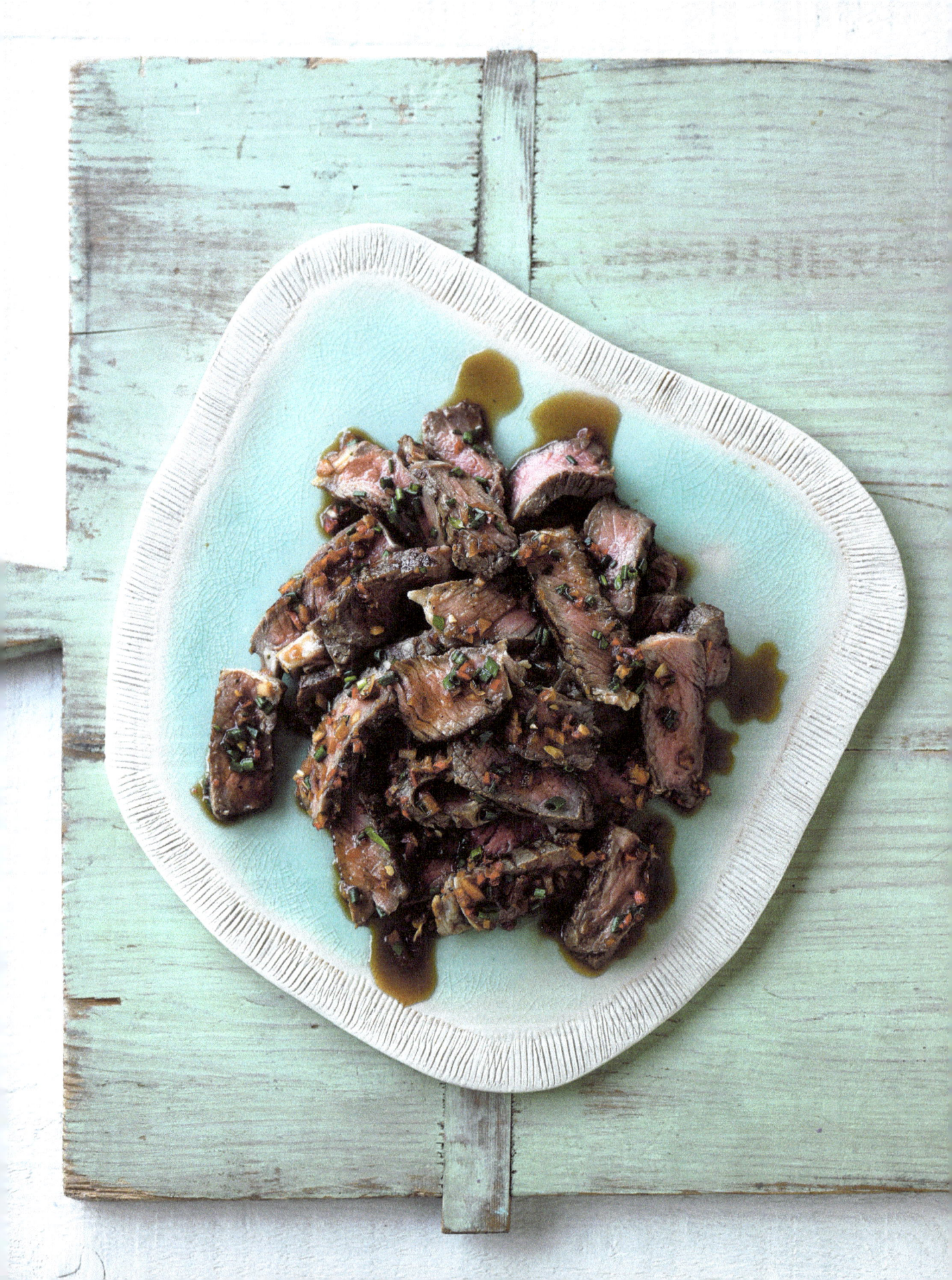

Adobo Beef

Time to prepare: 15 minutes
Time to cook: 6 minutes + 6 minutes to rest

SERVES: 6

6 x 300g beef sirloin steaks
¼ cup avocado oil
⅓ cup apple cider vinegar
¼ cup tamari
2 teaspoons freshly ground black pepper
1 clove garlic, peeled and crushed
2 fresh long red chilli, finely chopped
1 tablespoon 100% maple syrup
1 small red onion, peeled and finely chopped
1 small bunch fresh chives, thinly sliced

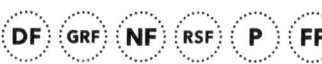

1. Season both sides of your steak with sea salt and freshly ground black pepper. Allow to come to room temperature.

2. Pop all of your remaining ingredients together in a glass or ceramic baking dish large enough so that your steaks will fit side by side in a single layer. Season with sea salt and freshly ground black pepper. Set the dressing mixture aside.

3. Preheat a large char-grill pan or barbecue char-grill plate to medium. Once hot, add your steaks. Char-grill, untouched (and I mean it here, do not poke or prod your steak with tongs, turn or lift slightly to see underneath and do not shuffle it around on your char-grill), for 3 minutes. Turn and char-grill, untouched again, for another 3 minutes for medium-rare.

4. Transfer your steak to the dressing mixture in your dish in a single layer. Stand for 3 minutes, then gently turn and stand for another 3 minutes until the meat has rested.

5. Remove your steak from the dressing to a chopping board and thickly slice against the grain. Return the sliced steak to the dressing mixture and toss gently to combine. Serve steak with the lovely dressing mixture spooned over.

HEALTHY MEALS

Beef Bourguignon

Time to prepare: 10 minutes
Time to cook: 6 minutes + 6 minutes to rest

1. Season both sides of your steak with sea salt and freshly ground black pepper. Allow to come to room temperature.

2. Pop all of your remaining ingredients together in a glass or ceramic baking dish large enough so that your steaks will fit side by side in a single layer. Season with sea salt and freshly ground black pepper. Set the dressing mixture aside.

3. Preheat a large char-grill pan or barbecue char-grill plate to medium. Once hot, add your steaks. Char-grill, untouched (and I mean it here, do not poke or prod your steak with tongs, turn or lift slightly to see underneath and do not shuffle it around on your char-grill), for 3 minutes. Turn and char-grill, untouched again, for another 3 minutes for medium-rare.

4. Transfer your steak to the dressing mixture in your dish in a single layer. Stand for 3 minutes, then gently turn and stand for another 3 minutes until the meat has rested. Serve steak with the lovely dressing mixture spooned over.

SERVES: 6

6 x 300g beef sirloin steaks
½ cup avocado oil
⅓ cup red wine vinegar
1 small bunch fresh flat-leaf parsley, leaves finely chopped
½ small bunch fresh thyme, leaves picked
1 clove garlic, peeled and crushed
4 small eschallots, peeled and very thinly sliced
4 slices pancetta, very thinly sliced
50g button mushrooms, very thinly sliced

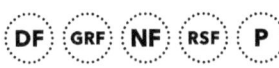

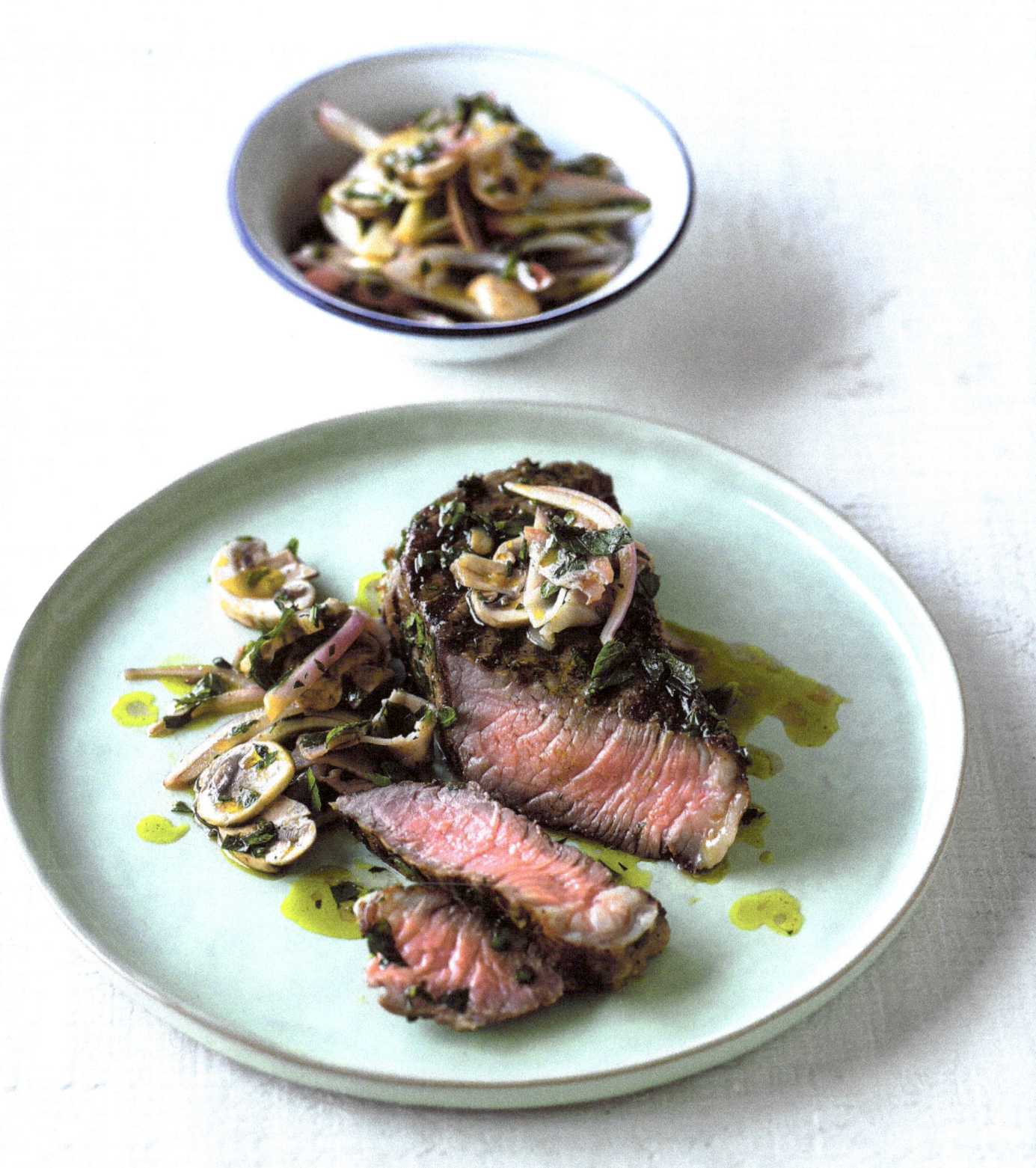

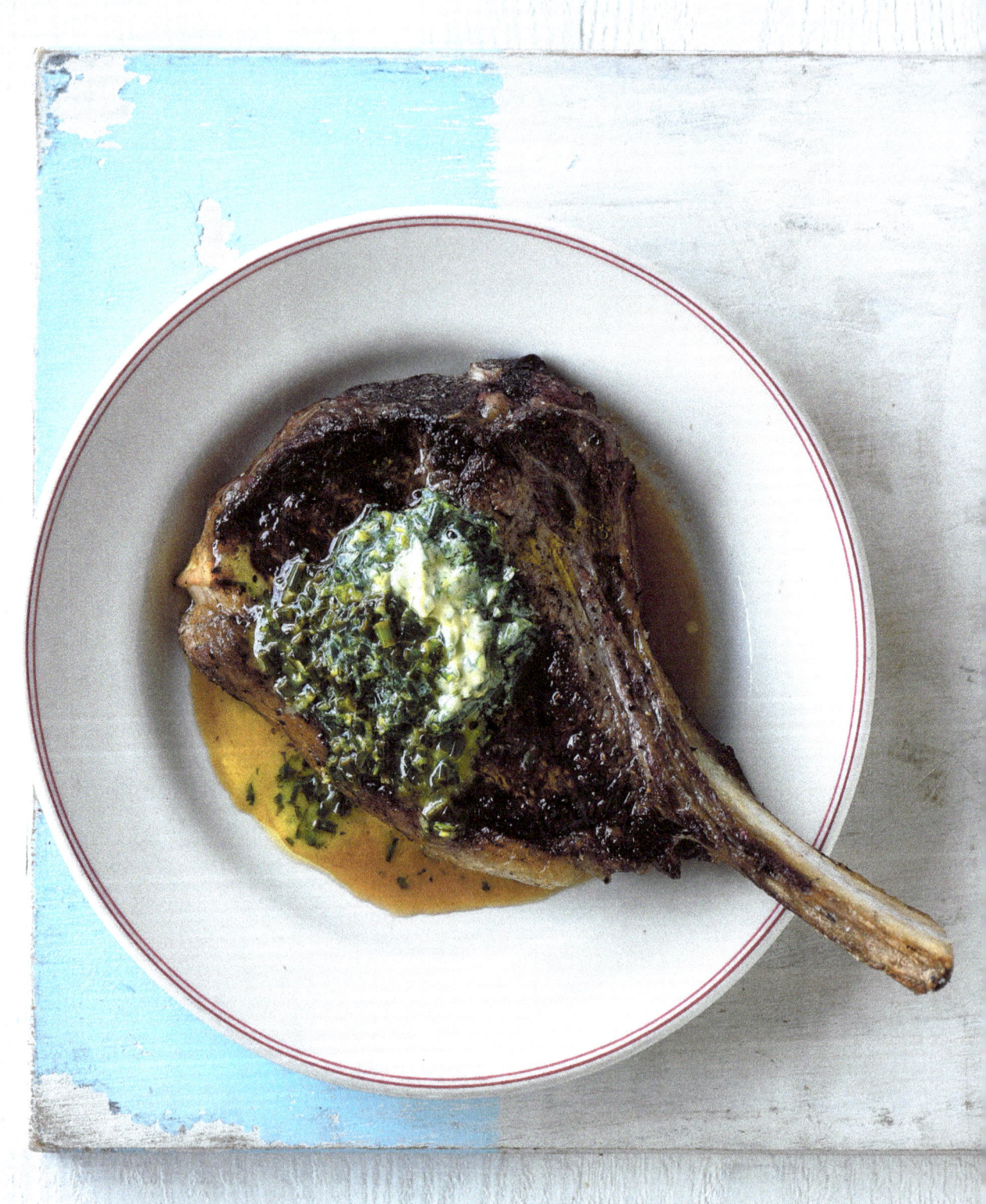

Meat-lovers Rib-eye

Time to prepare: 10 minutes
Time to cook: 14 minutes + 5 minutes to rest

1. Season both sides of your steak with sea salt and freshly ground black pepper. Allow to come to room temperature.

2. Preheat your oven to 200°C/180°C fan-forced. Line a large baking tray with non-stick baking paper.

3. Pop all of your remaining ingredients together in a bowl and stir well to combine. Season with sea salt and freshly ground black pepper. Set the butter mixture aside.

4. Preheat a large char-grill pan or barbecue char-grill plate to medium. Once hot, add your steaks. Char-grill, untouched (and I mean it here, do not poke or prod your steak with tongs, turn or lift slightly to see underneath and do not shuffle it around on your char-grill), for 3 minutes. Turn and char-grill, untouched again, for another 3 minutes for medium-rare.

5. Transfer your steak to the prepared tray and bake for 8 minutes for medium-rare or cook until your liking. Remove from the oven and stand for 5 minutes until the meat has rested. Serve steak with the lovely butter mixture dolloped on top.

SERVES: 6

6 x 400g beef rib-eye cutlets
80g butter, at room temperature
2 large lemons, zest finely grated and then juiced
1 small bunch fresh flat-leaf parsley, leaves finely chopped
1 small bunch fresh chives, thinly sliced

(GRF) (NF) (RSF) (P) (FF)

- HAZELNUTS
- BABY KALE LEAVES
- LEBANESE CUCUMBER
- BABY CHARD LEAVES
- BABY SPINACH LEAVES
- MICRO RADISH
- BLOOD ORANGE
- GREEN BEANS
- BRUSSELS SPROUTS
- FLAXSEED OIL
- MICRO ROCKET

salad sides

Roasted Cauliflower & Pomegranate / *108*
Heirloom Tomato Salad / *111*
Spring Salad / *112*
Baby Greens Salad / *115*
Super-green Slaw / *116*
Winter Citrus & Thyme Salad / *119*

ALL ABOUT SALAD SIDES

Who says salads are just for spring and summer? I don't! Enjoy these warm and cold variations all-year-round. They are a great way of adding extra nutrient dense vegetables and fruits into your everyday meals. Simply mix and match these vibrant salads with any of the meals in this cookbook.

Roasted Cauliflower & Pomegranate

Time to prepare: 15 minutes + 30 minutes standing time
Time to cook: 30 minutes

1. Preheat your oven for a good 15 minutes to 200°C/180°C fan-forced. Line a large baking tray with non-stick baking paper.

2. Place your cauliflower on the prepared tray in a single layer. Combine your butter, coriander and sweet paprika in a small bowl, then brush over both sides of the cauliflower. Roast for 20 minutes, turn the cauliflower slices, then roast for another 10 minutes or until tender and golden.

3. Meanwhile, combine your onion and vinegar in a bowl and stand at room temperature for 30 minutes, turning occasionally, or until the onion softens and releases its lovely pink colour into the vinegar.

4. Arrange your warm roasted cauliflower, baby kale and pickled onion onto a serving platter and then sprinkle with the pomegranate seeds. Serve warm.

SERVES: 6

1 head of cauliflower, untrimmed and thickly sliced crosswise
50g butter, melted
1 teaspoon ground coriander
1 teaspoon sweet paprika
1 large red onion, peeled and very thinly sliced into rings
⅓ cup apple cider vinegar
50g baby kale leaves
1 pomegranate, seeds released (see note)

(GRF) (NF) (RSF) (P) (V)

RECIPE NOTE

The easiest way to release the seeds from a fresh pomegranate is to slice the fruit in half then place a half, cut side facing down, into your palm and wrap your fingers around to hold firmly, then use a rolling pin or large wooden spoon to strongly tap the skin of the fruit which will release all the seeds. Be sure to have a large bowl placed underneath your hand to catch all the seeds and any delicious juice.

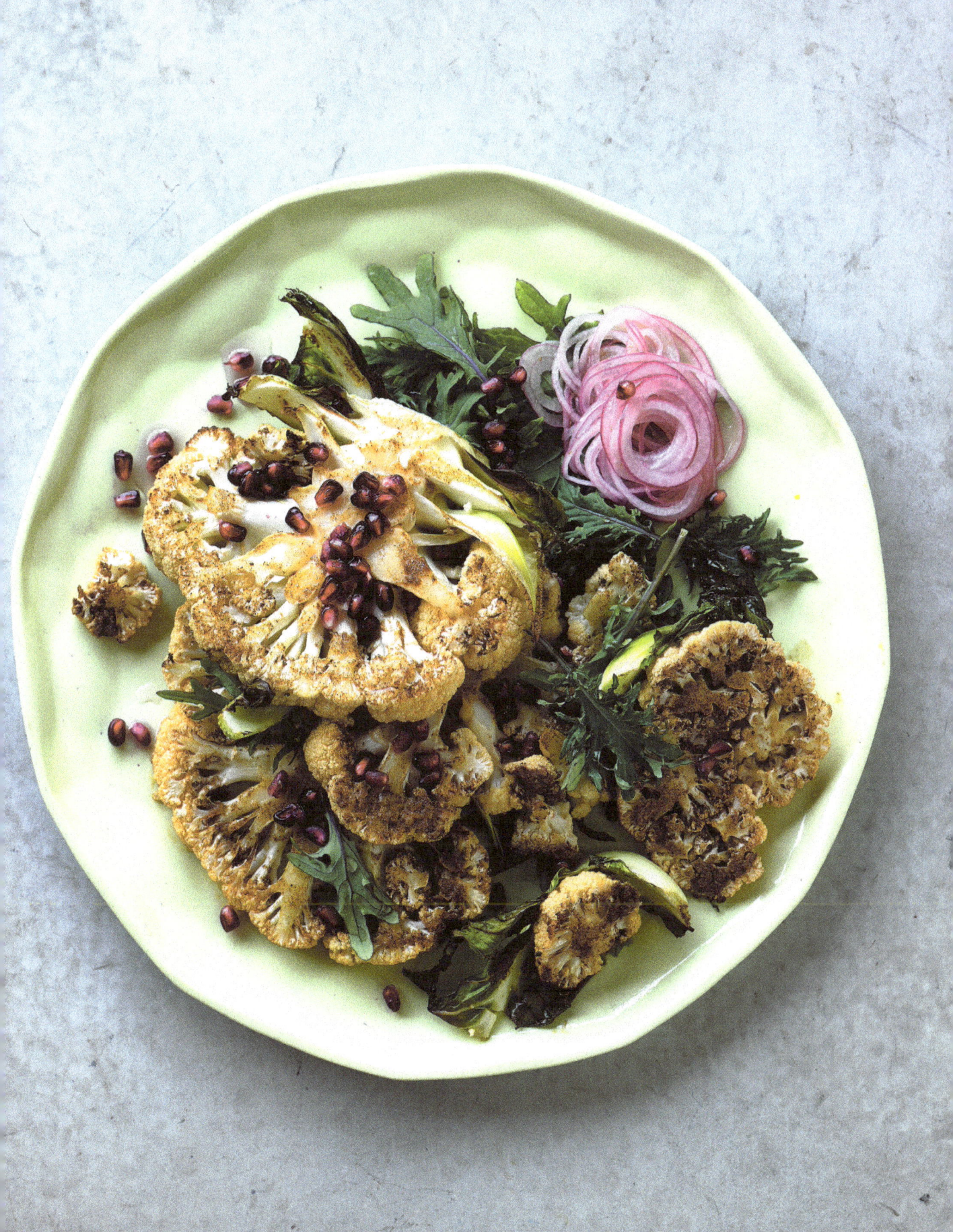

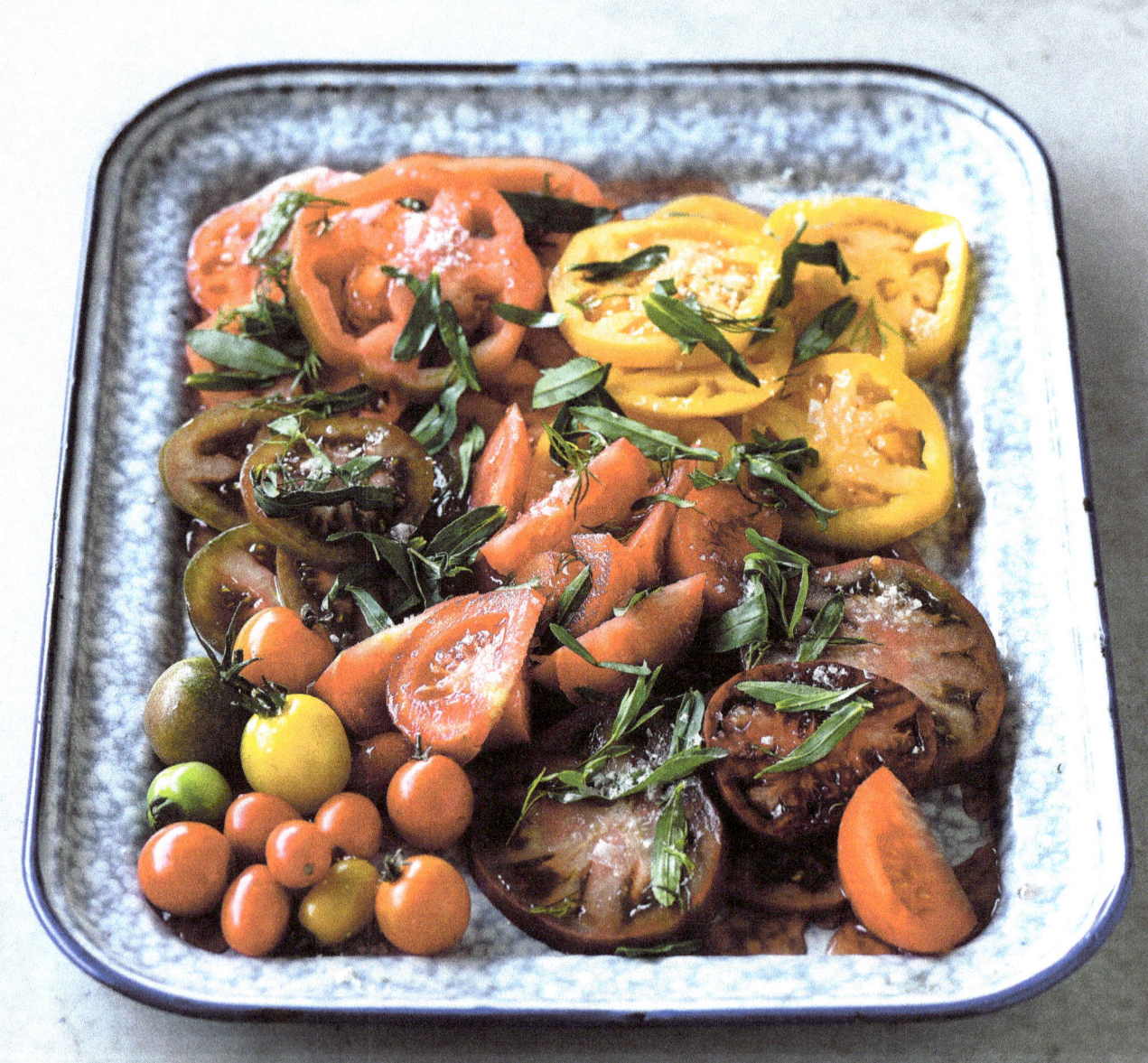

Heirloom Tomato Salad

Time to prepare: 10 minutes + 20 minutes standing time

1. Place your vinegar, syrup and tomato into a large bowl. Season with freshly ground black pepper. Toss very gently together and cover with a tea towel. Stand at room temperature, giving it a gentle toss occasionally, for 20 minutes or until all of the natural juice begins to release from the tomato.
2. Transfer your tomato to a serving platter and sprinkle with your tarragon, dill and sea salt. Serve.

SERVES: 6

¼ cup red wine vinegar

3 teaspoons 100% maple syrup

600g mixed heirloom tomatoes, small ones left whole, larger ones sliced into rounds or cut into wedges

1 small bunch fresh tarragon, leaves picked

½ small bunch fresh dill, leaf tips picked

3 teaspoons pink sea salt

(DF) (GRF) (NF) (RSF) (P) (VG)

Spring Salad

Time to prepare: 15 minutes

1. Make Tracey's Dressing first by placing all of the ingredients into a screw top jar and season with sea salt and freshly ground black pepper. Screw the jar's lid on tightly, then shake vigorously until well combined. Stand at room temperature.

2. Place your asparagus, fennel, green bean, cucumber and parsley into a large bowl, then gently toss together to combine. Season with sea salt and freshly ground black pepper. Transfer to a serving plate, then drizzle with Tracey's Dressing. Sprinkle with your pepitas. Serve.

SERVES: 6

2 bunches green asparagus, woody ends trimmed and thinly sliced diagonally
3 baby fennel, trimmed and very thinly sliced lengthwise
100g green beans, trimmed and thinly sliced into rounds
2 Lebanese cucumbers, thinly sliced into rounds
1 small bunch flat-leaf parsley, leaves picked
¼ cup pepitas (shelled pumpkin seeds)

TRACEY'S DRESSING

¼ cup flaxseed oil
2 tablespoons apple cider vinegar
2 tablespoons maple syrup
3 teaspoons brown mustard seeds

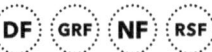

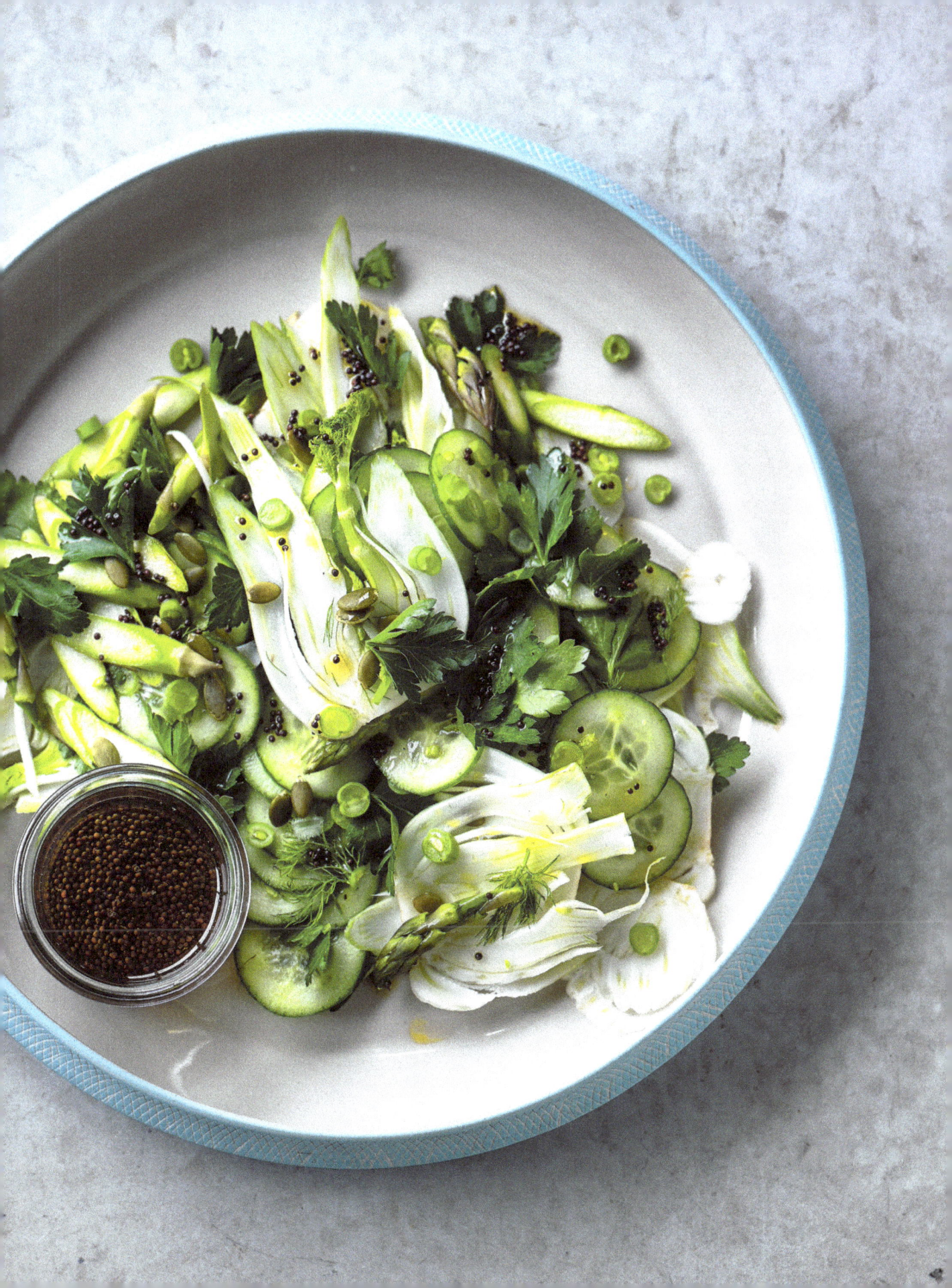

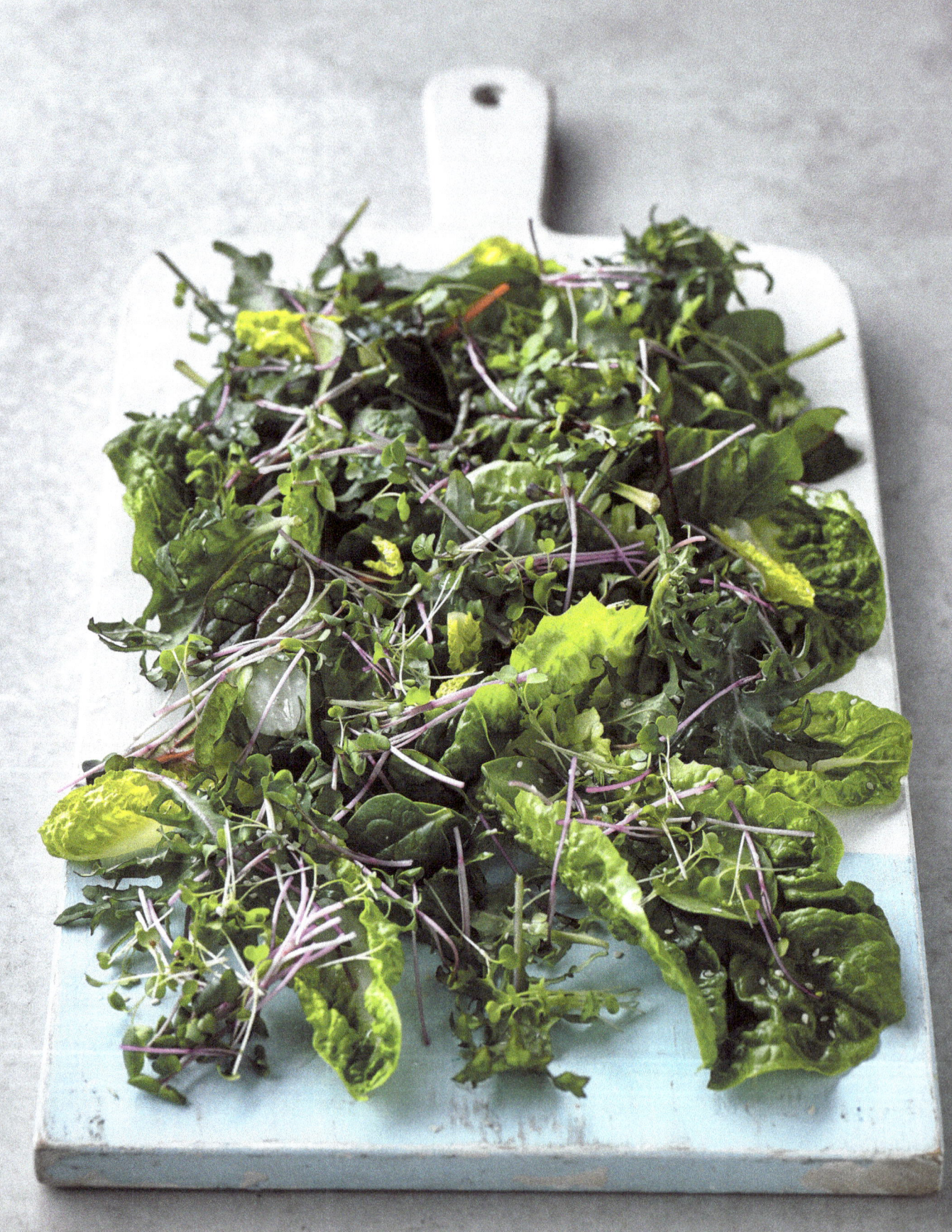

Baby Greens Salad

Time to prepare: 10 minutes

1. Place all of your ingredients into a large bowl and toss gently to combine. Arrange your salad onto a large chopping board or serving platter. Serve.

RECIPE NOTE

You can purchase punnets of micro herbs from farmers markets, green grocers, and large supermarkets. Use can use any combination of varieties available.

SERVES: 6

50g mixed baby leaves (kale, chard and spinach)
1 baby cos, leaves separated
1 punnet micro rocket, snipped from punnet base (see note)
1 punnet micro radish, snipped from punnet base (see note)
2 teaspoons sesame seeds
1 lime, juiced

HEALTHY MEALS

Super-green Slaw

Time to prepare: 10 minutes

1. Place your avocado oil and orange juice into a large bowl, then whisk until well combined. Season with sea salt and freshly ground black pepper.

2. Add all of your remaining ingredients to the bowl, then toss gently to combine. Arrange your salad onto a serving plate. Serve.

SERVES: 6

¼ cup avocado oil
1 small orange, juiced
1 bunch English spinach, leaves picked and thinly shredded
¼ iceberg lettuce, thinly shredded
6 Brussels sprouts, trimmed and very thinly sliced
½ cup hazelnuts, chopped

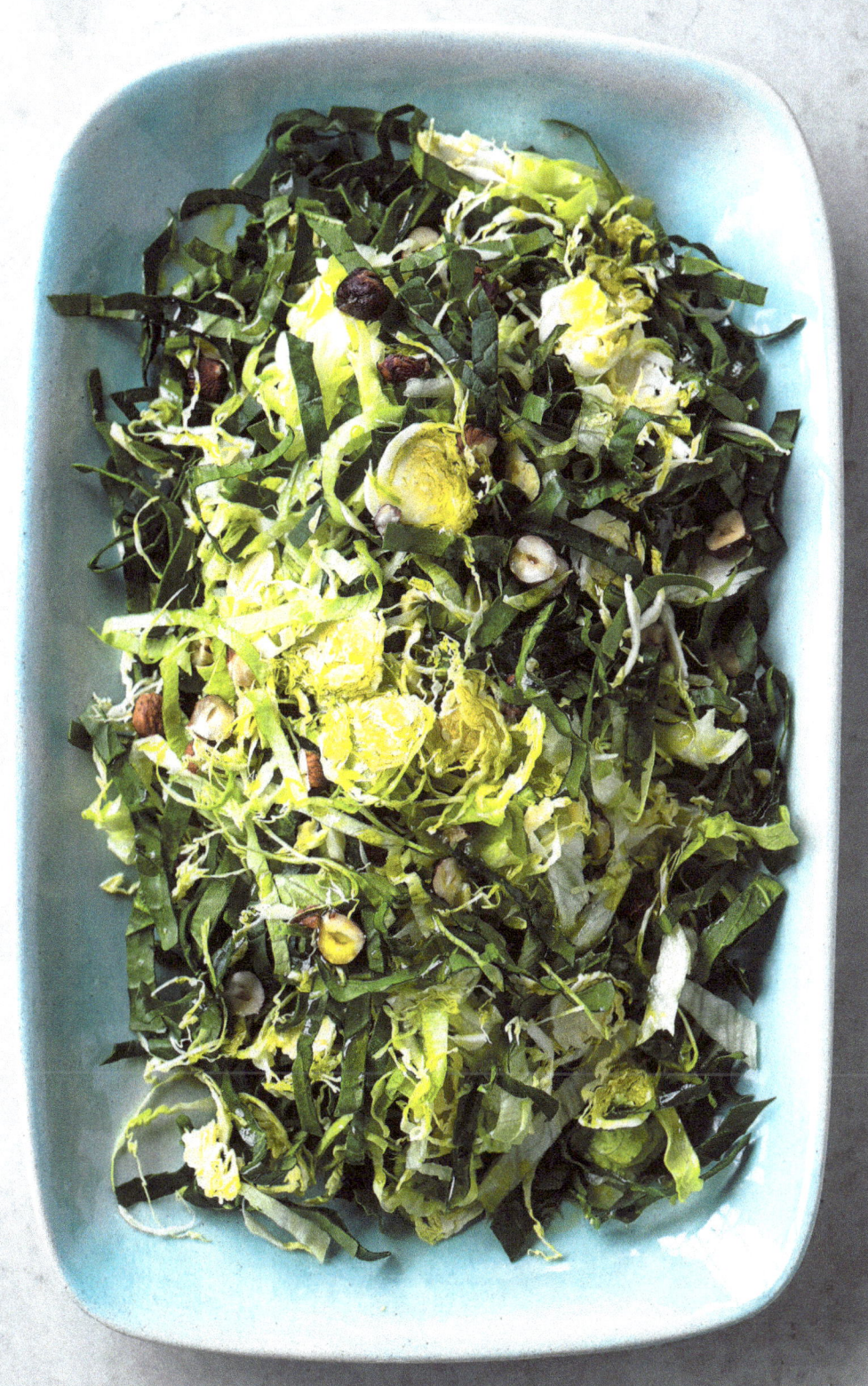

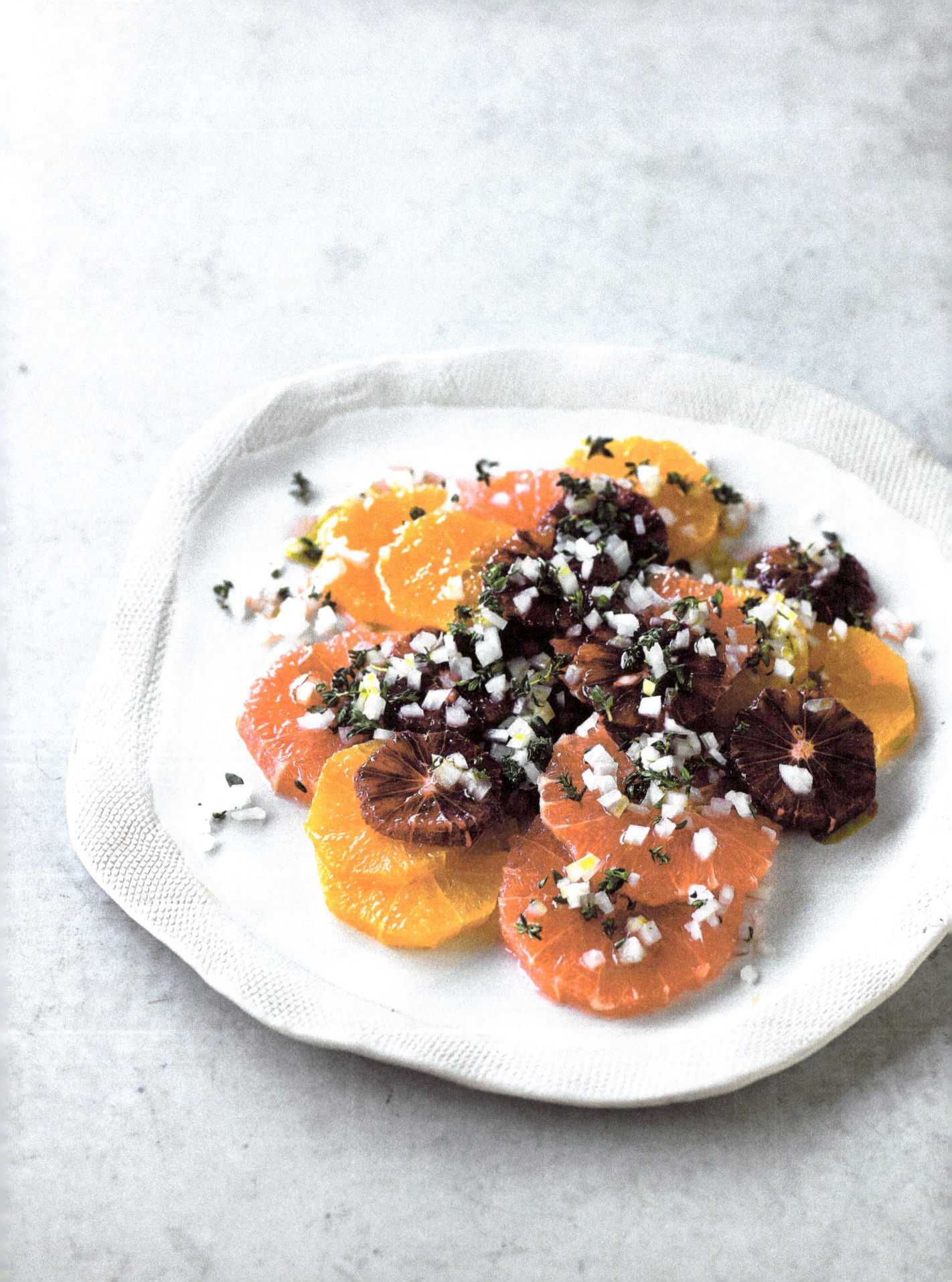

Winter Citrus & Thyme Salad

Time to prepare: 10 minutes

1. Arrange your citrus onto a serving platter.
2. Place your thyme and onion together in a bowl, then toss gently to combine. Sprinkle the mixture over your citrus, then drizzle with your avocado oil. Serve.

RECIPE NOTE

Be sure to catch and keep any of the citrus juice that escapes on peeling and slicing and then drizzle it over your salad before serving.

SERVES: 6

1 ruby grapefruit, peeled and sliced into thin rounds
2 oranges, peeled and sliced into thin rounds
4 blood oranges, peeled and sliced into thin rounds
½ small bunch fresh thyme, leaves picked
1 small white onion, peeled and finely chopped
1 tablespoon avocado oil

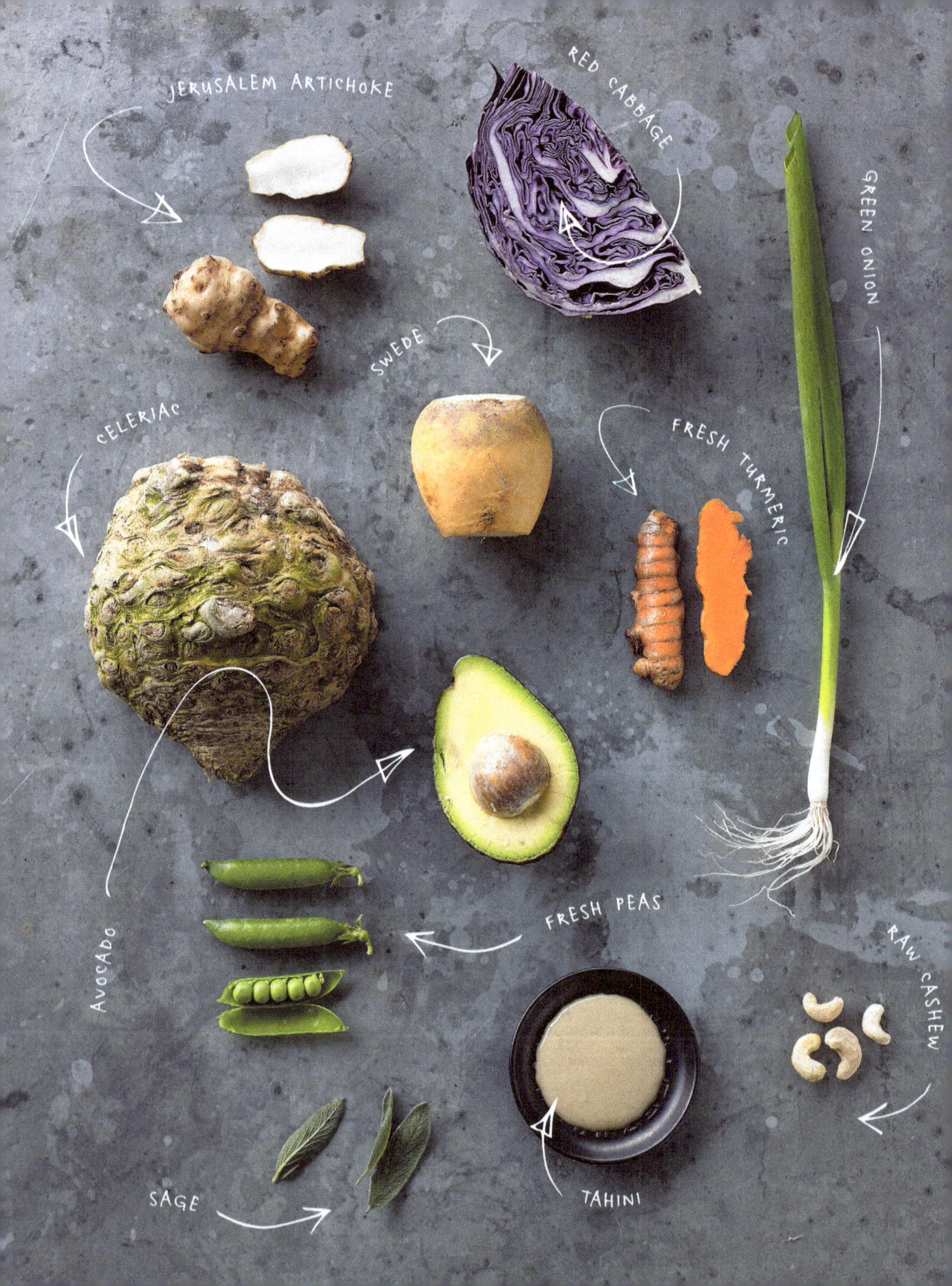

JERUSALEM ARTICHOKE

RED CABBAGE

GREEN ONION

SWEDE

CELERIAC

FRESH TURMERIC

AVOCADO

FRESH PEAS

RAW CASHEW

SAGE

TAHINI

smash sides

Whipped Sweet Potato Chump / *125*

Carrot & Swede Colcannon / *126*

Smoky Summer Eggplant / *129*

Artichoke & Celeriac / *130*

Roast Pumpkin & Sage Brown Butter / *133*

Zesty Avocado & Pea / *134*

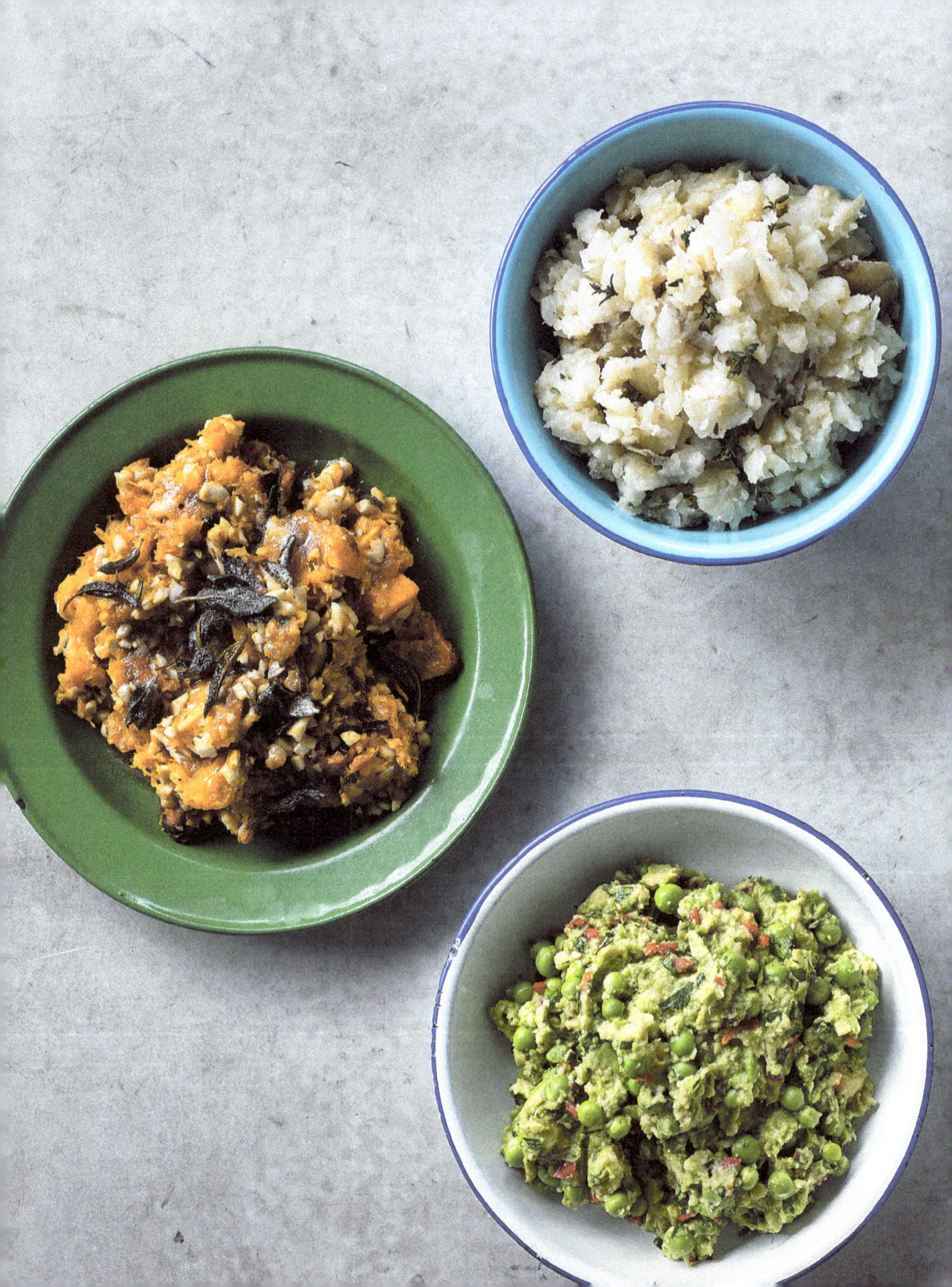

ALL ABOUT SMASH SIDES

A 'smash' – is basically the consistency of a chunky mash and all I use is a fork to produce them.

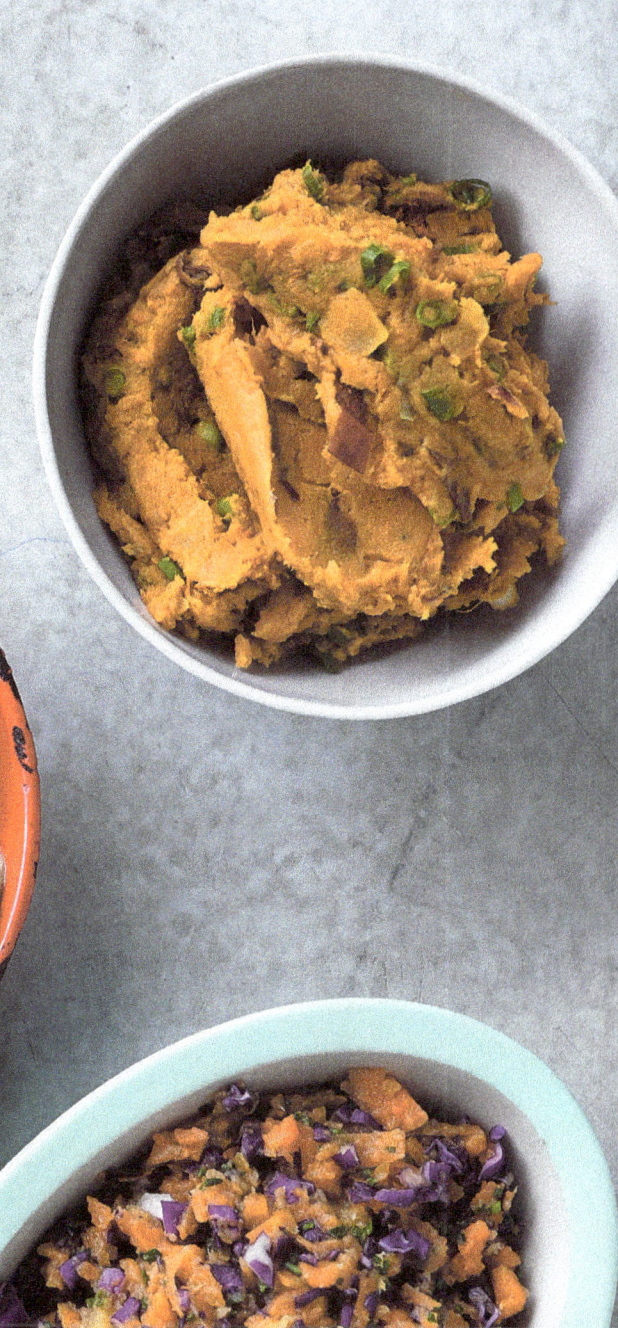

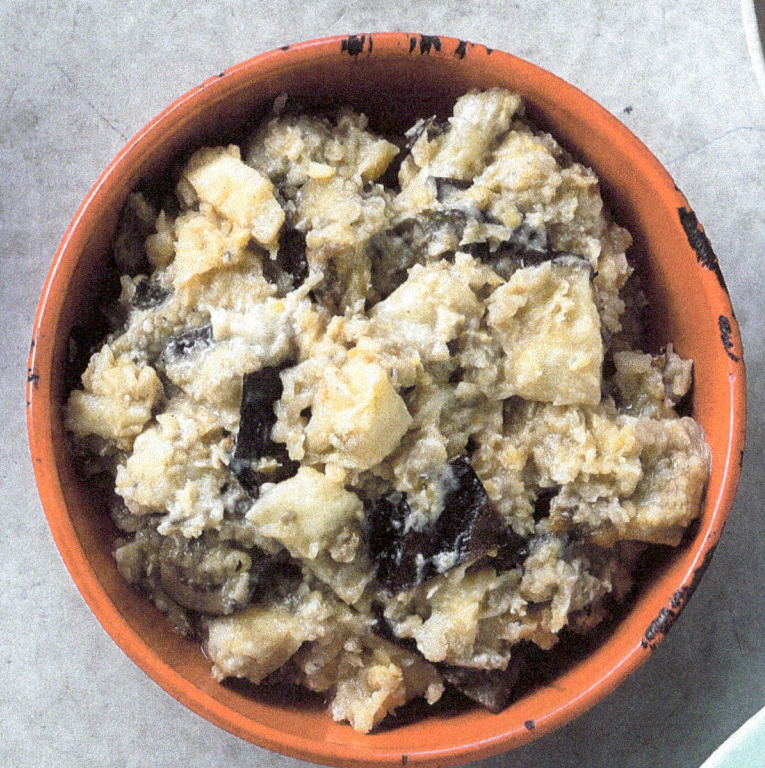

It's part of my genetic Irish heritage that makes me crave a good 'smash' quite regularly which is why I've dedicated a chapter to my favourite combos.

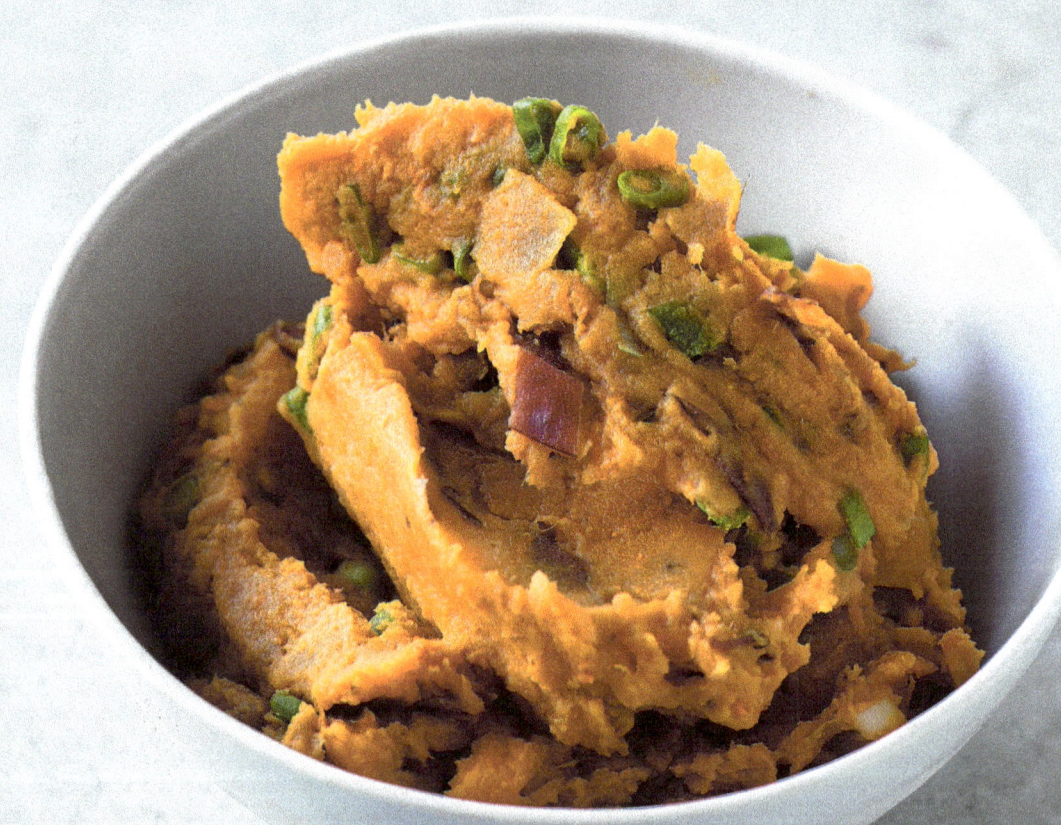

Whipped Sweet Potato Chump

Time to prepare: 15 minutes
Time to cook: 17 minutes

1. Steam your sweet potato for 15 minutes or until tender. Transfer your sweet potato to a large heat proof bowl and mash lightly with a fork to break apart the pieces.

2. Preheat a small saucepan over a medium heat. Add your butter and swirl the pan occasionally until it melts. Stir in your green onion and cook, stirring constantly, for 2 minutes or until tender but not coloured. Transfer the butter mixture to the bowl with the sweet potato.

3. Using a hand held electric whisk, whisk the mixture together until really smooth and fluffy. Add your turmeric, then stir until well combined. Season with sea salt and freshly ground black pepper. Serve.

SERVES: 6

600g orange sweet potato, chopped
50g butter
4 green onions, thinly sliced
2cm piece fresh turmeric, finely grated

Carrot & Swede Colcannon

Time to prepare: 10 minutes
Time to cook: 15 minutes

1. Steam your carrot and swede together for 15 minutes or until tender. Transfer your vegetables to a large heatproof bowl and mash well with a fork to as smooth as you like.
2. Add your butter, cabbage and chives to the bowl, then stir until your butter melts and mixture is well combined. Season with sea salt and freshly ground black pepper. Serve.

SERVES: 6

2 large carrots, chopped
1 swede, peeled and chopped
25g butter
100g red cabbage, finely chopped
1 small bunch fresh chives, thinly sliced

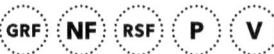

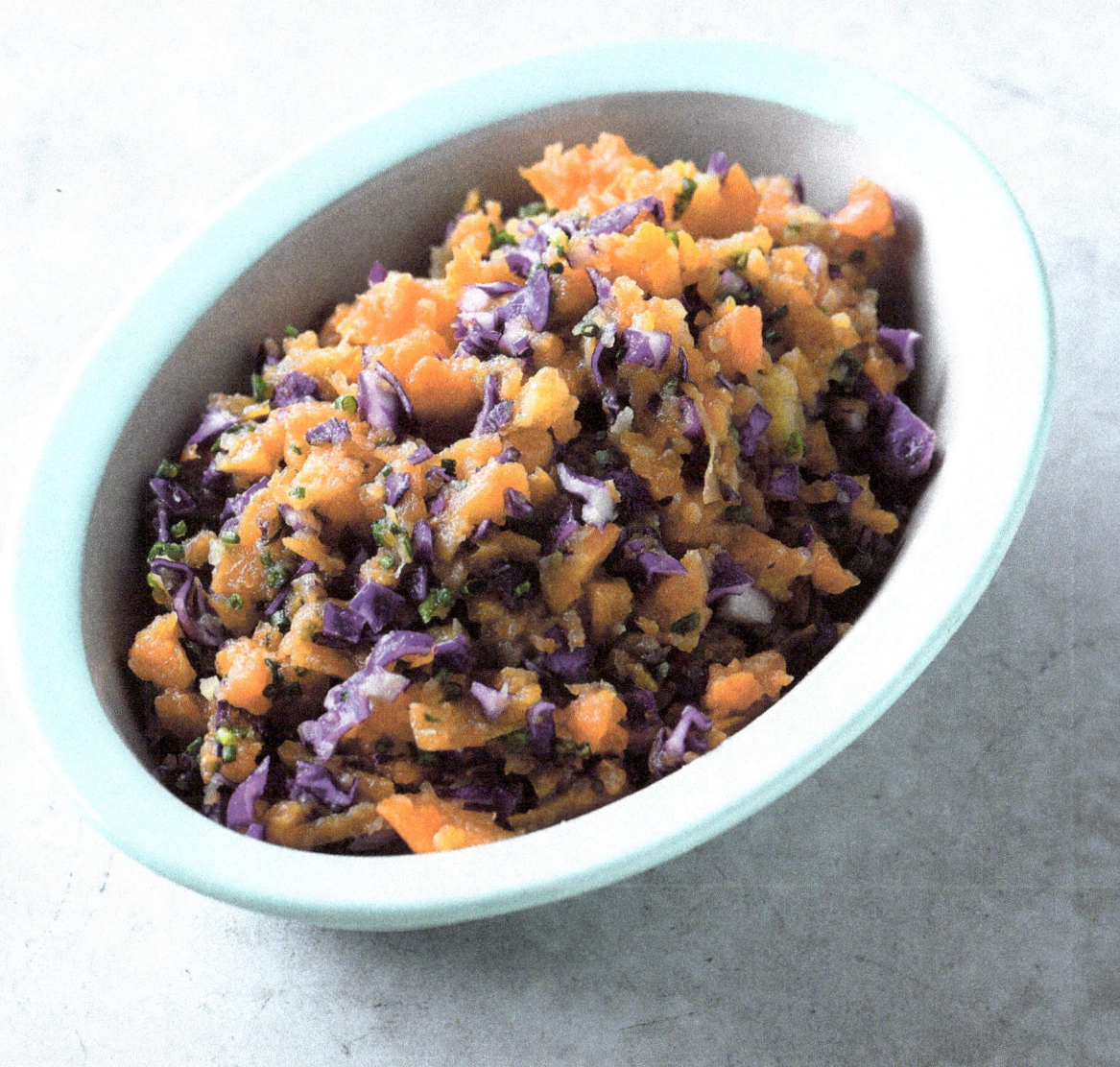

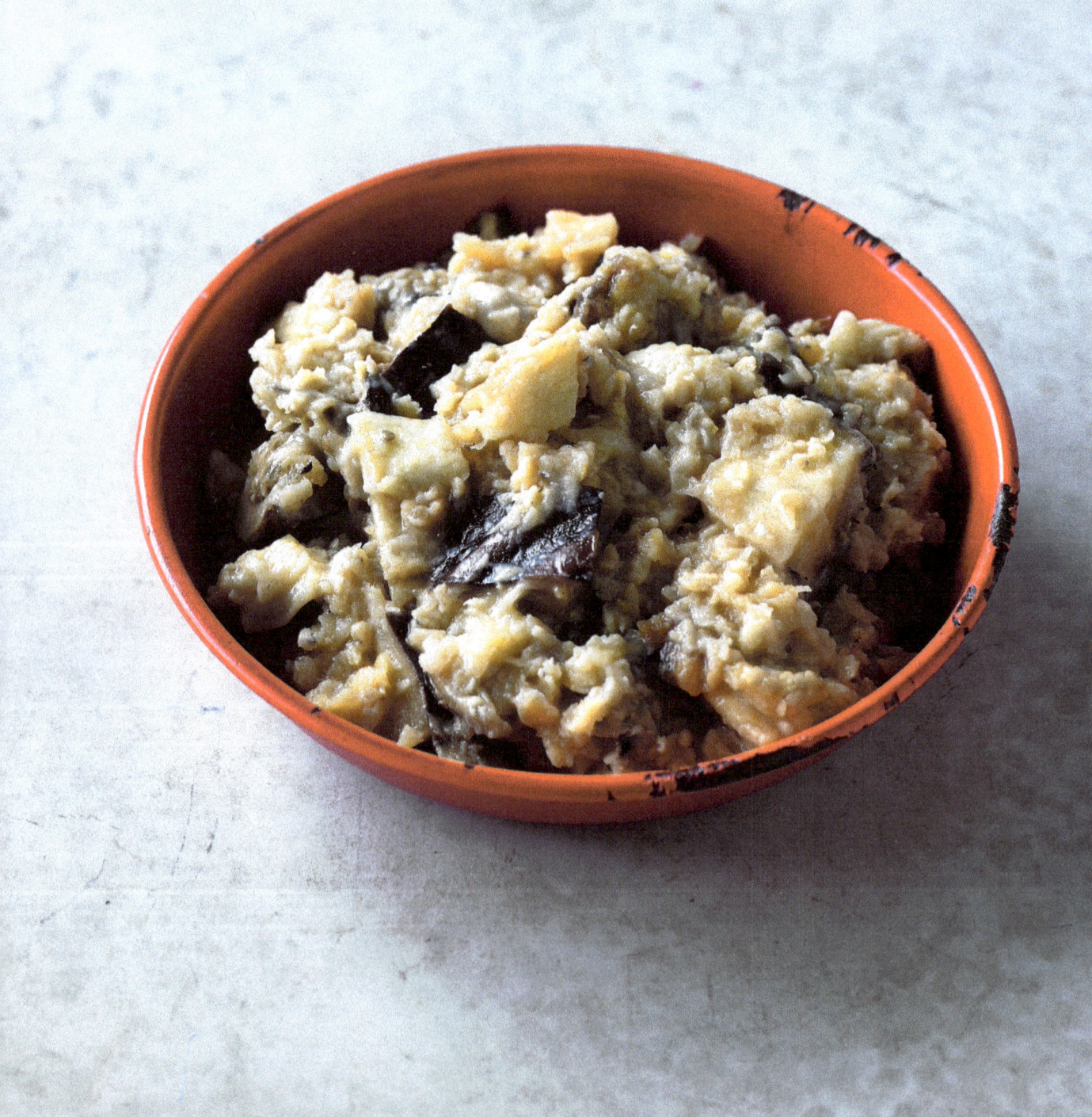

Smoky Summer Eggplant

Time to prepare: 10 minutes
Time to cook: 15 minutes + 5 minutes resting

1. Place your lentils into a small saucepan and cover with cold water. Place your saucepan over a high heat and cook, stirring occasionally, for 15 minutes or until the lentils are tender. Drain very well, then transfer your lentils to a large heatproof bowl.

2. Meanwhile, heat a large char-grill pan or barbecue char-grill plate on high. Add your eggplant and char-grill, turning occasionally, for 15 minutes or until the skin has blistered and the eggplant flesh feels tender when gently pierced with a fork. Transfer your eggplant to a chopping board and rest for 5 minutes, then trim and discard the ends. Roughly chop your eggplant then scoop up and add to the bowl with the lentils.

3. Add all of your remaining ingredients to the bowl, then stir until well combined. Season with sea salt and freshly ground black pepper. Serve.

SERVES: 6

¾ cup dried split red lentils
1 large eggplant
1 clove garlic, peeled and crushed
2 tablespoons macadamia oil
1 tablespoon tahini
1 lemon, zest finely grated and juiced

DF **GRF** **RSF** **P** **VG**

Artichoke & Celeriac

Time to prepare: 10 minutes
Time to cook: 20 minutes

1. Steam your artichoke and celeriac for 20 minutes or until tender. Transfer your vegetables to a large heatproof bowl and mash well with a fork to as smooth as you like.

2. Add all of your remaining ingredients to the bowl, then stir until your butter melts and mixture is well combined. Season with sea salt and freshly ground black pepper. Serve.

SERVES: 6

500g Jerusalem artichokes, chopped
300g celeriac, peeled and chopped
25g butter
½ small bunch fresh thyme, leaves picked

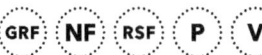

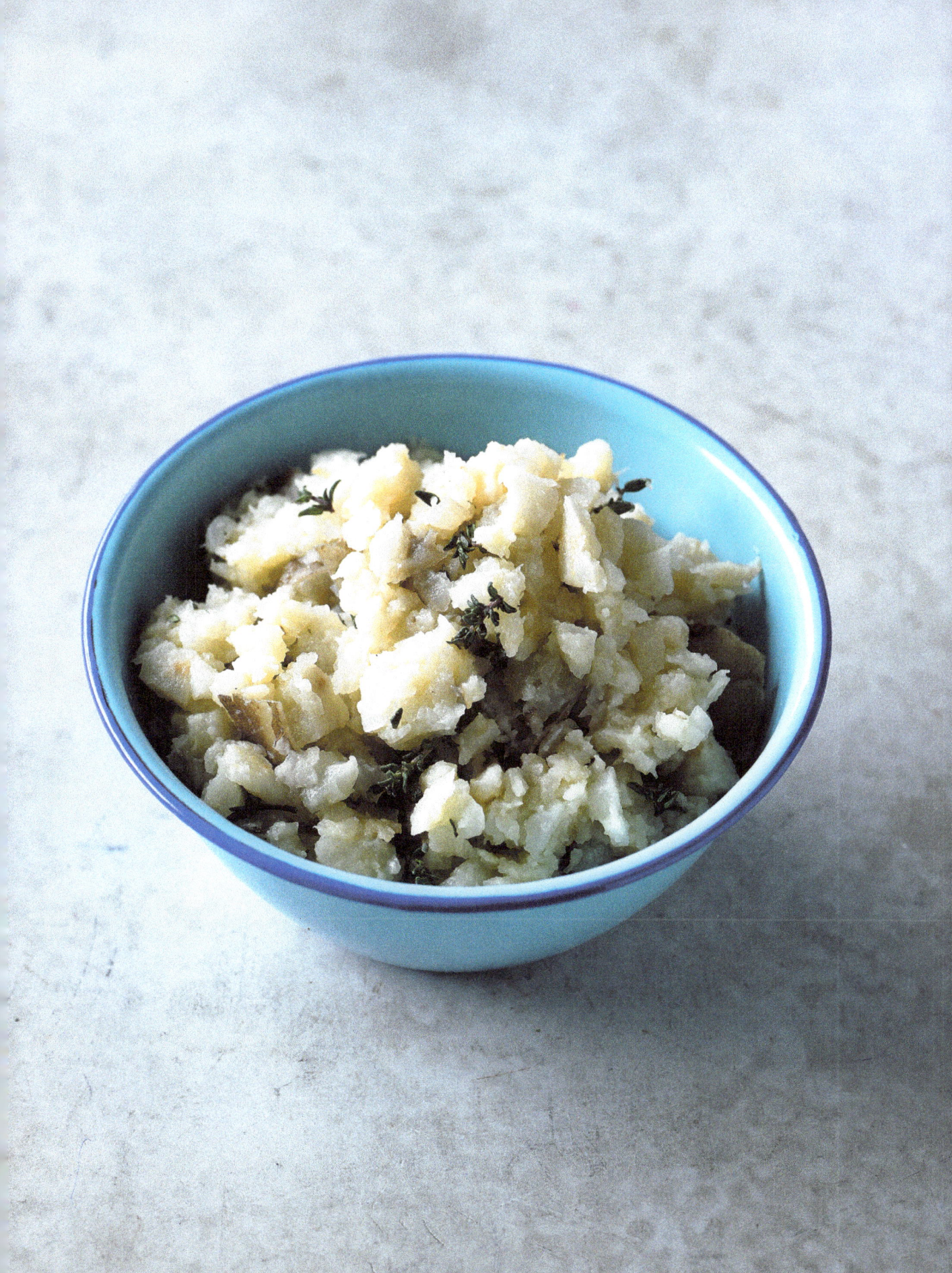

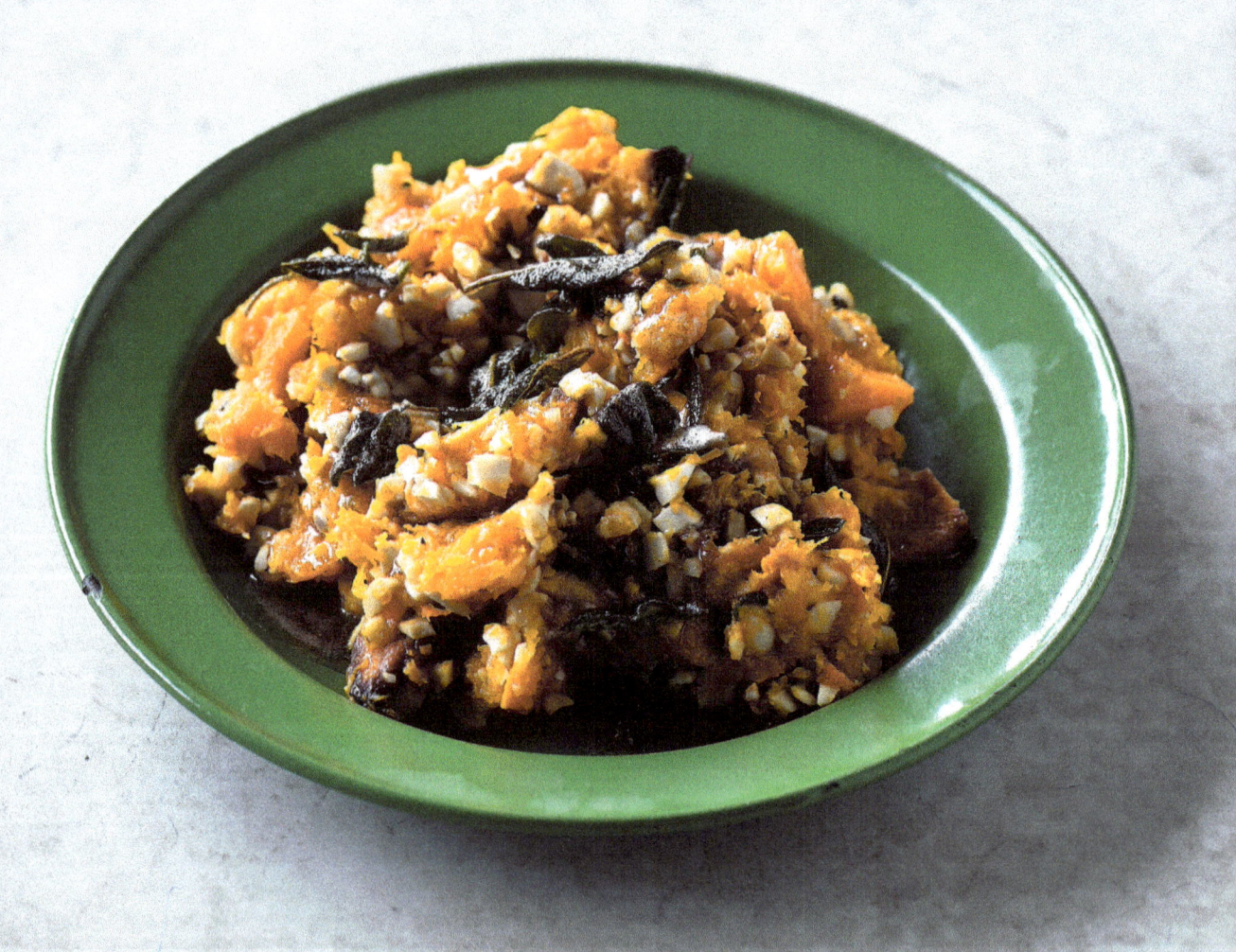

Roast Pumpkin & Sage Brown Butter

Time to prepare: 20 minutes
Time to cook: 27 minutes

1. Preheat your oven for a good 15 minutes to 200°C/180°C fan-forced. Line a large baking tray with non-stick baking paper.
2. Place your pumpkin onto the prepared tray, drizzle with your honey and then dot with your coconut oil. Roast for 25 minutes or until tender and golden. Transfer to a large heatproof bowl and mash well with a fork to as smooth as you like.
3. Meanwhile, place your cashew into a heatproof bowl and cover with boiling water. Stand for 15 minutes to soften slightly, then drain and rinse under cold running water. Chop as finely as possible.
4. Preheat a small frying pan over a medium heat. Add your butter and sage and swirl the pan occasionally for 2 minutes or until the butter melts, becomes foamy, turns to a nut brown colour and the sage becomes crisp. Pour the butter mixture into the bowl with the pumpkin, add the finely chopped cashew, then stir until mixture is well combined. Season with sea salt and freshly ground black pepper. Serve.

SERVES: 6

600g peeled and seeded butternut pumpkin, chopped
2 teaspoons honey
1 tablespoon coconut oil
½ cup raw cashews
50g butter
1 small bunch fresh sage, leaves picked

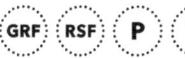

Zesty Avocado & Pea

Time to prepare: 10 minutes

1. Place your avocado into a large bowl and mash well with a fork to as smooth as you like.
2. Add all of your remaining ingredients to the bowl, then stir until well combined. Season with sea salt and freshly ground black pepper. Serve.

RECIPE NOTE

You can also use frozen peas if fresh are unavailable, simply pop them onto a large plate that has a few pieces of kitchen paper towel on top and allow to thaw to room temperature before using. You can even add them in partially frozen as I do sometimes, the children love it and it also gives a lovely crunch to the smash.

SERVES: 6

- 3 avocados, halved, stones removed and flesh scooped out from skin
- 1 lime, zest finely grated and juiced
- 1 long red chilli, finely chopped
- ¼ cup flat-leaf parsley leaves, finely chopped
- ¾ cup shelled fresh peas (see note)

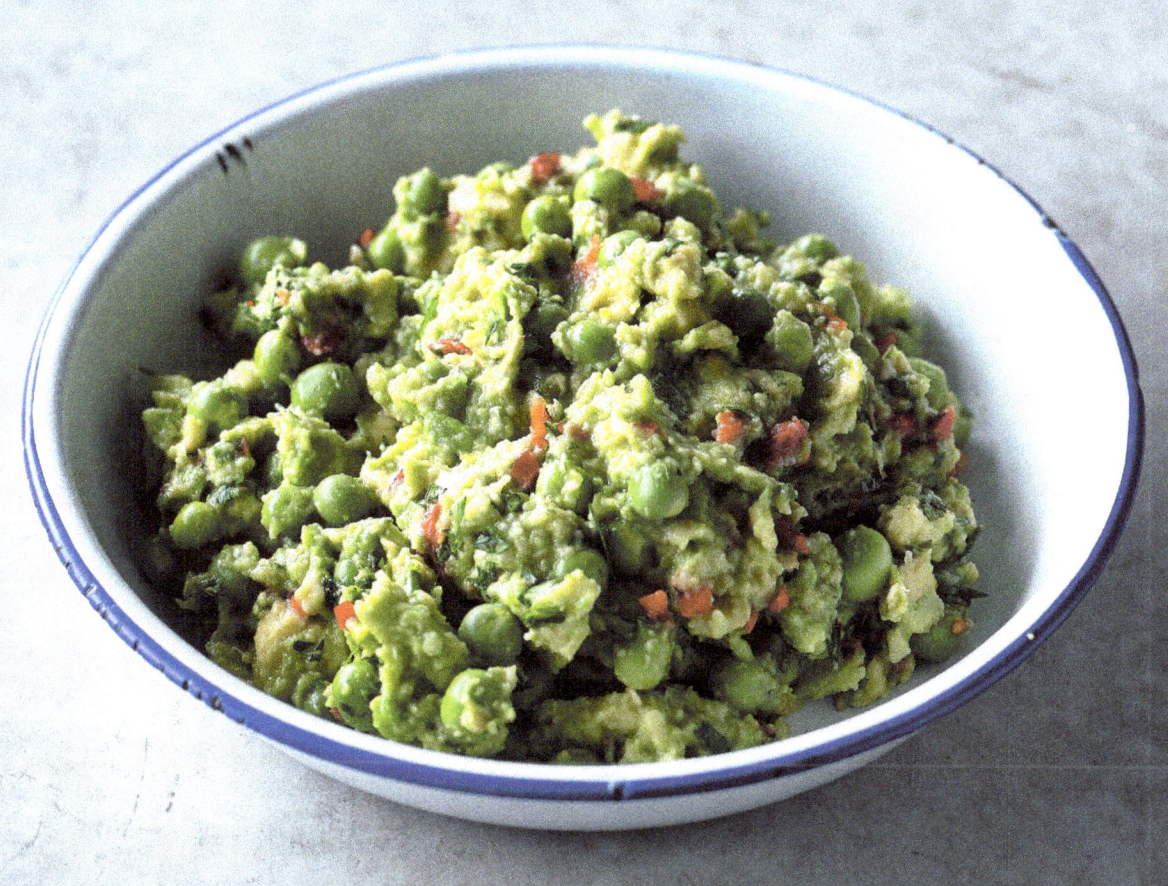

- BROCCOLINI
- BEETROOT
- BABY TURNIP
- BABY PARSNIP
- MACADAMIA OIL
- CORIANDER SEEDS
- SWISS BROWN MUSHROOM
- OYSTER MUSHROOMS
- ENOKI MUSHROOM
- CUMIN SEEDS
- SHITAKE MUSHROOM
- KING BROWN MUSHROOM

vege sides

Mushrooms with Crispy Chilli & Ginger / *141*
Winter Bake / *142*
Raw Peas with Macadamia / *145*
Glazed Beets & Sprouts / *146*
Braised Cabbage / *149*
Blistered Capsicum & Tomato / *150*

ALL ABOUT VEGE SIDES

It is really important to fill at least half of your plate with a rainbow of colour from fresh produce at every meal to ensure you are getting an abundant amount of nutrients on a daily basis. I cook the following vege sides for weekly family meals and for special occasions. They are the perfect flavour additions to any meal.

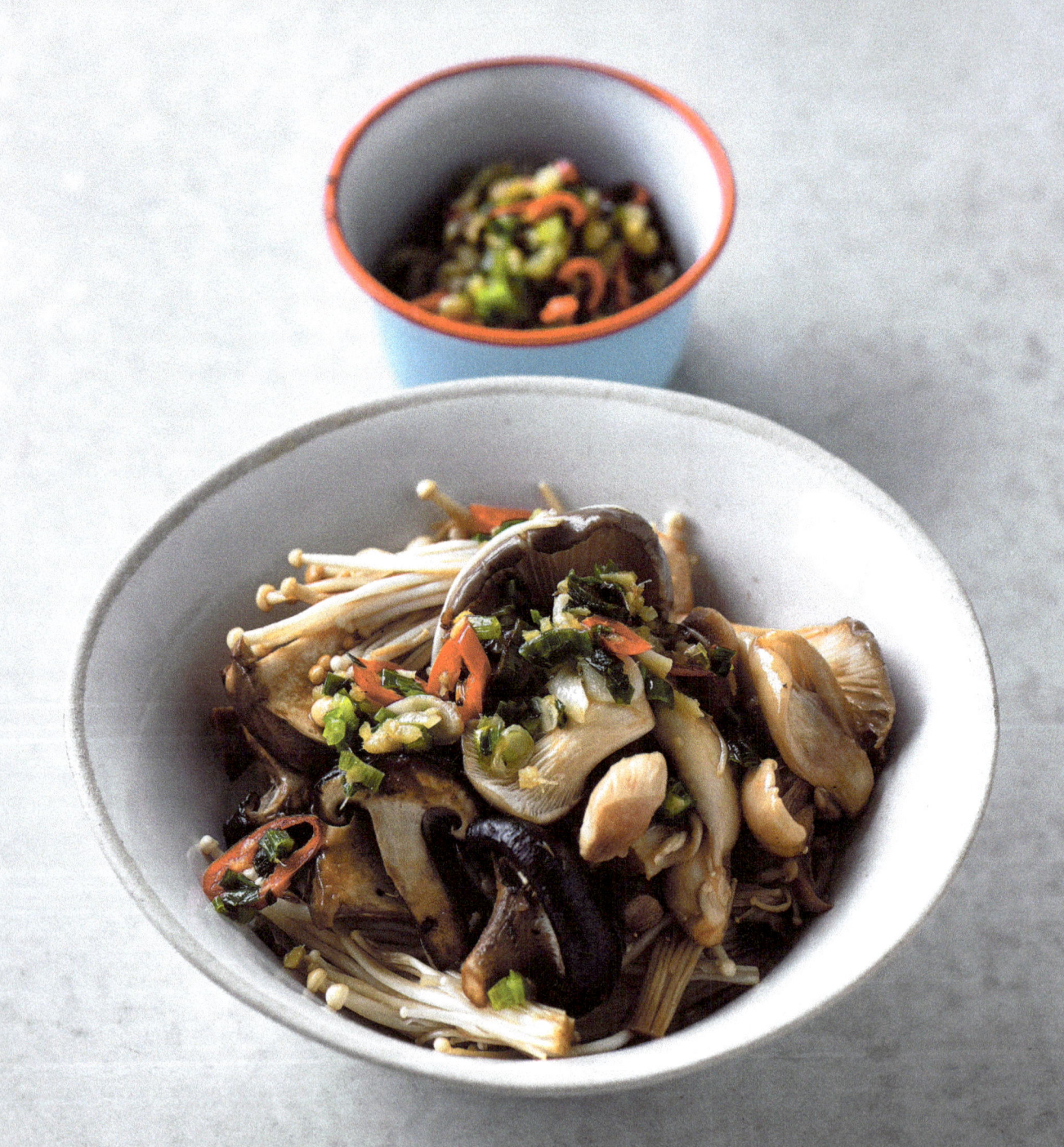

Mushrooms with Crispy Chilli & Ginger

Time to prepare: 10 minutes
Time to cook: 4 minutes

1. Preheat your wok over a high heat. Add your coconut oil and swirl the wok until melted. Add your chilli, ginger, green onion and garlic and stir-fry for 2 minutes or until crispy and golden. Using a slotted spoon (you want to keep the oil in the wok) transfer the crispy chilli mixture to a heatproof bowl.

2. Reheat the same wok over a high heat. Add all your remaining ingredients and stir-fry for 2 minutes or until mushrooms are just tender. Transfer to a serving bowl, then sprinkle with the crispy chilli mixture. Serve.

SERVES: 6

1 tablespoon coconut oil
2 long red chilli, thinly sliced
4cm piece fresh ginger, peeled and finely chopped
4 green onions, thinly sliced
4 cloves garlic, peeled and thinly sliced
600g mixed mushrooms (oyster, enoki, shitake, Swiss brown, king brown), trimmed and left whole or torn in half
2 tablespoons tamari

(DF) (GRF) (NF) (RSF) (P) (VG)

Winter Bake

Time to prepare: 15 minutes
Time to cook: 30 minutes

1. Preheat your oven for a good 15 minutes to 200°C/180°C fan-forced.

2. Place your parsnip and turnip into a roasting pan and dot with the coconut oil. Season with sea salt and freshly ground black pepper. Bake for 20 minutes then remove from oven.

3. Add all of your remaining ingredients to the roasting pan, then toss until well combined. Bake for another 10 minutes or until vegetables and pear are just tender and golden. Serve.

SERVES: 6

6 baby parsnips, trimmed and halved lengthwise
240g baby turnips
1 tablespoon coconut oil
1 broccolini, trimmed and halved diagonally crosswise
1 green pear, cut into wedges and seeds removed
30g butter
2 cloves garlic, peeled and thinly sliced
½ small bunch fresh thyme, leaves picked

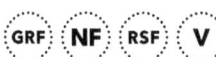

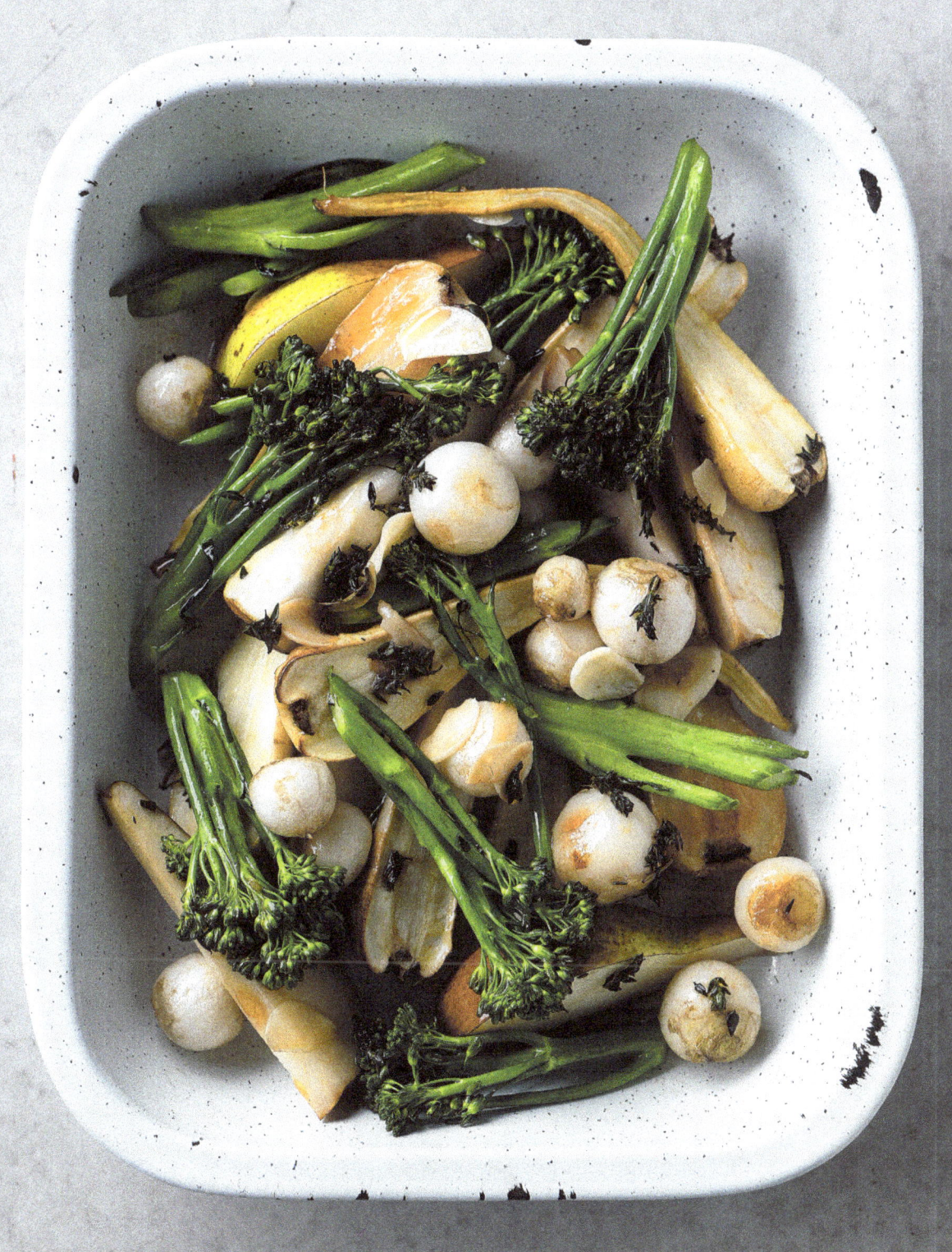

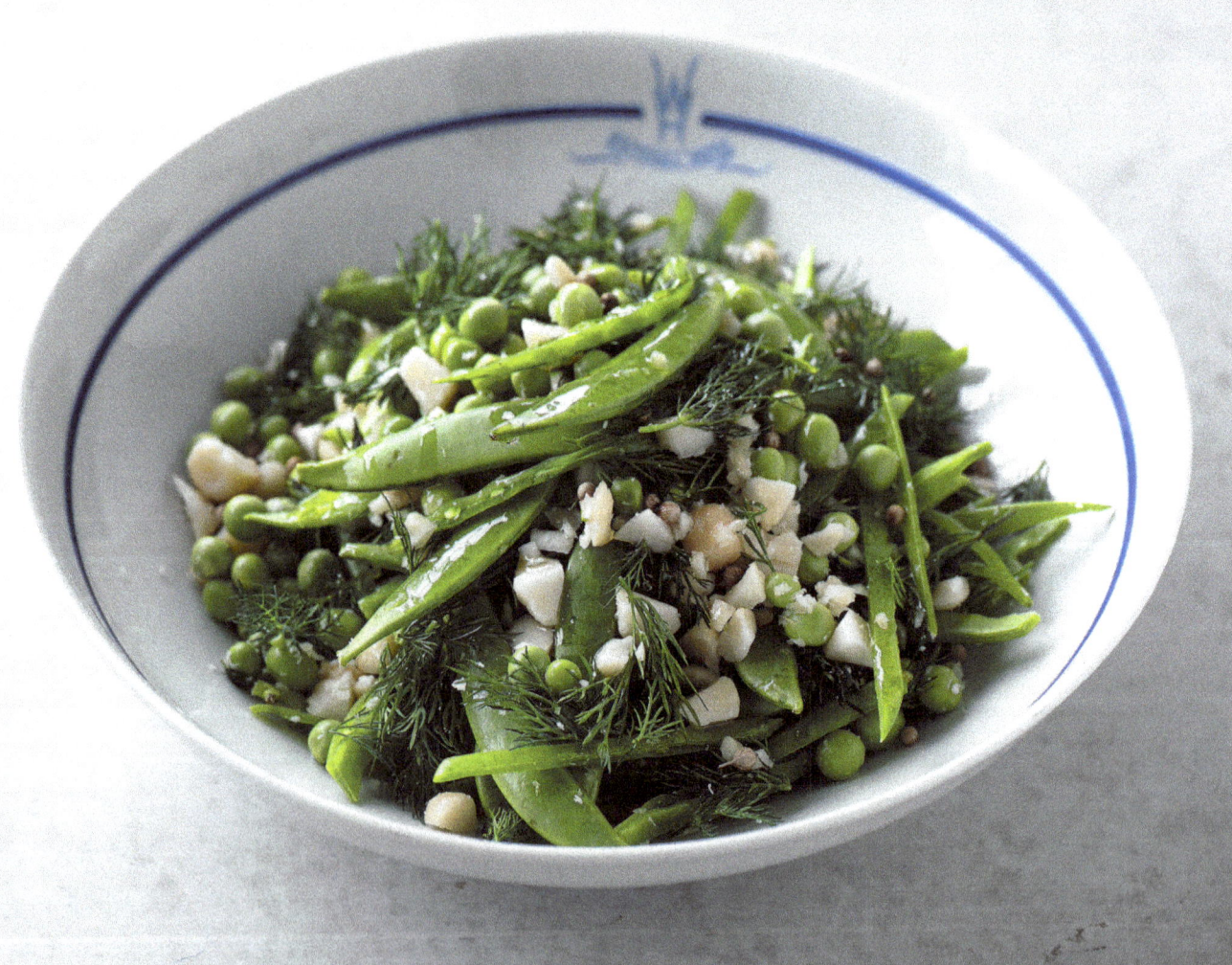

Raw Peas with Macadamia

Time to prepare: 10 minutes

1. Place all of your ingredients together in a large bowl, then toss gently until well combined. Arrange your salad onto a serving plate. Serve.

SERVES: 6

300g sugar snap peas, trimmed
300g snow peas, trimmed and thinly sliced lengthwise
1 cup shelled fresh peas
1 small bunch fresh dill, leaf tips picked
¼ cup raw macadamias, chopped
2 teaspoons coriander seeds, toasted and lightly crushed
2 tablespoons macadamia oil

Glazed Beets & Sprouts

Time to prepare: 10 minutes
Time to cook: 12 minutes

1. Steam your beetroot for 15 minutes or until almost tender.

2. Preheat a large, deep frying pan over a medium heat. Add your butter and swirl the pan until melted. Stir in your syrup and vinegar and once bubbling, add your beetroot and sprouts.

3. Cook, carefully turning the vegetables, for 5 minutes or until they are both tender. Stir through your salt, then transfer the vegetables to a serving plate. Serve.

SERVES: 6

4 small beetroot, trimmed and quartered lengthwise
50g butter
1 tablespoon 100% maple syrup
2 tablespoons apple cider vinegar
400g small Brussels sprouts, trimmed and halved lengthwise
2 teaspoons sea salt

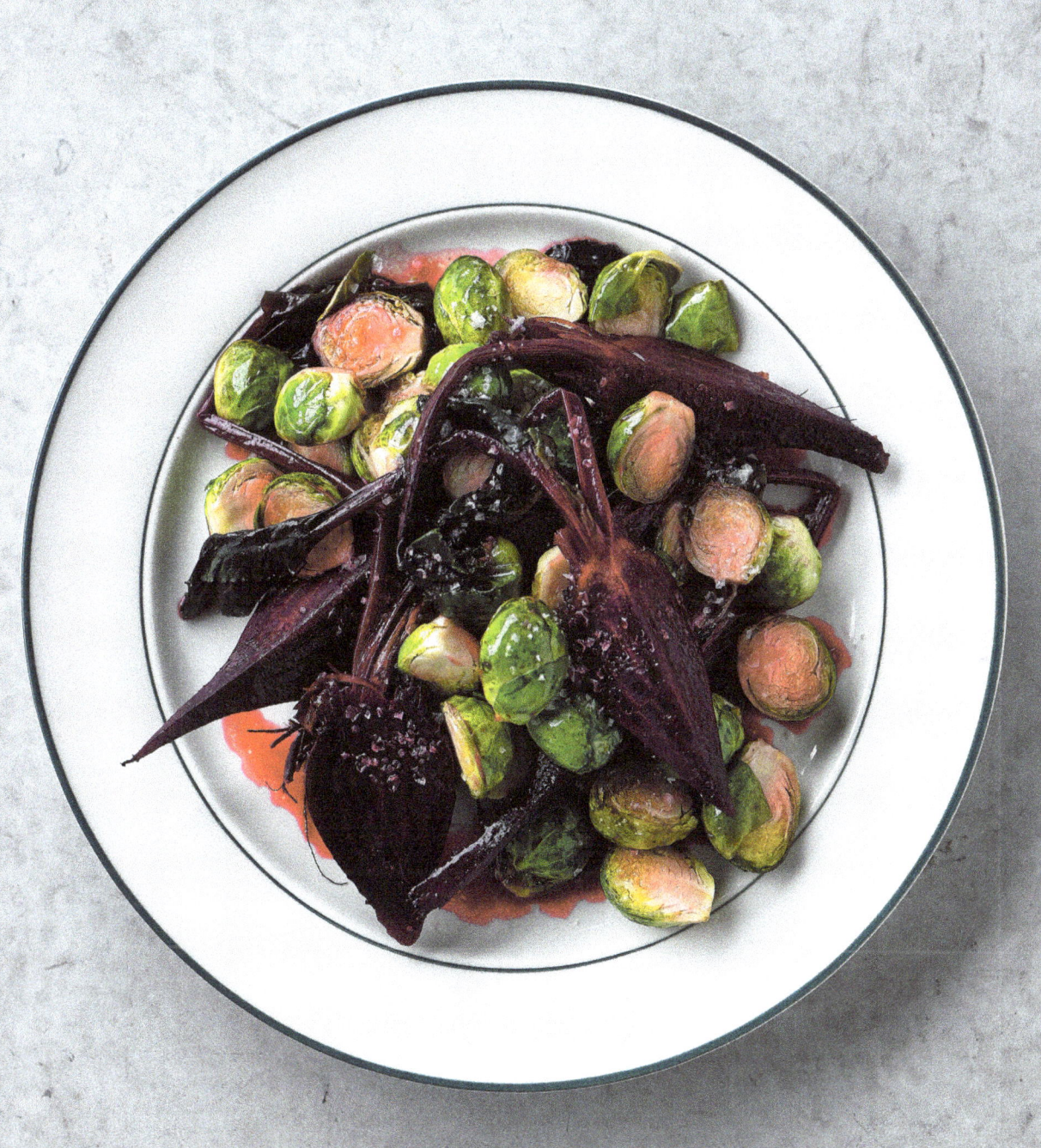

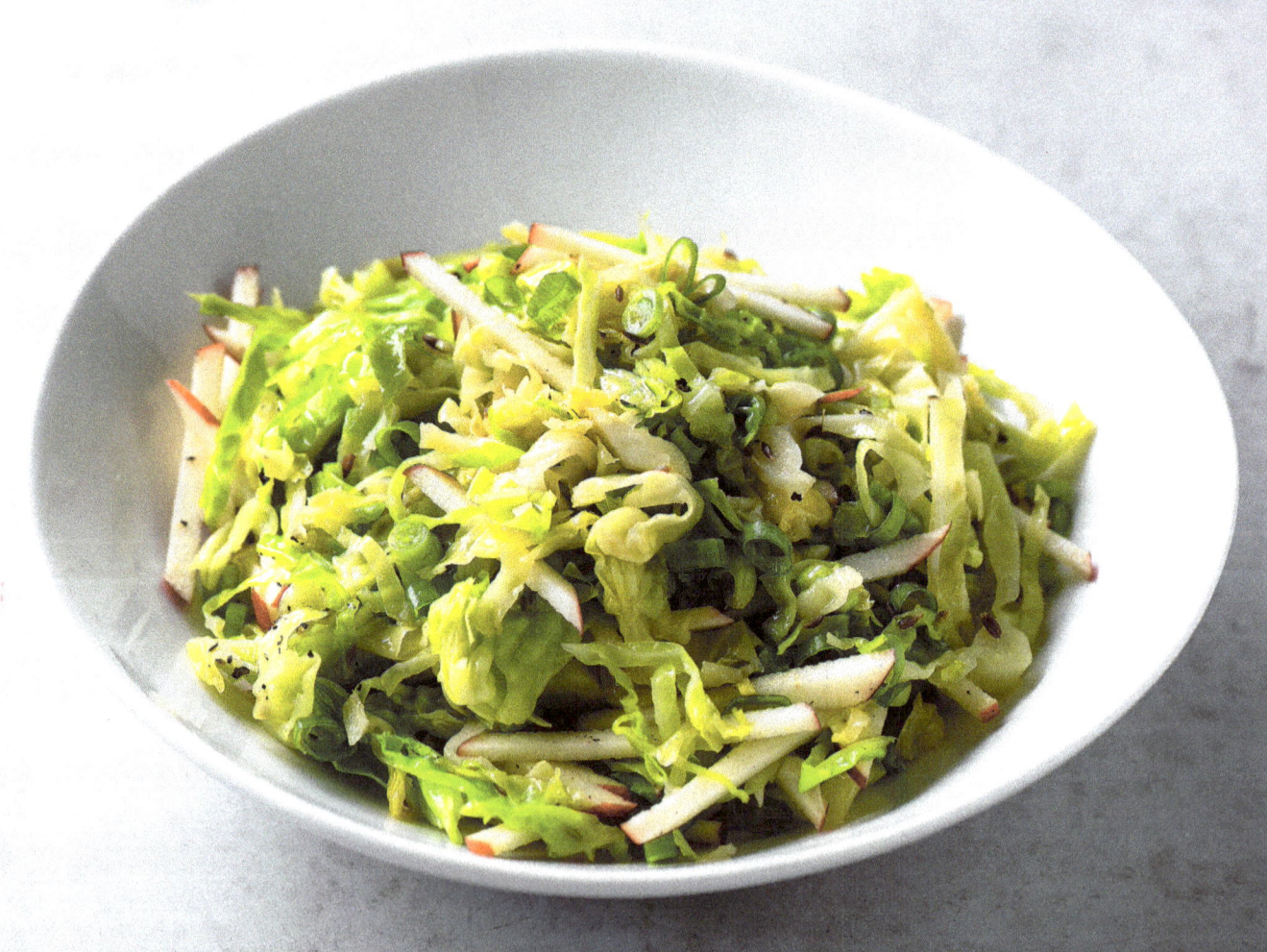

Braised Cabbage

Time to prepare: 10 minutes
Time to cook: 16 minutes

1. Preheat a large saucepan over a medium heat. Add your butter and swirl the pan until melted. Add the cumin seed and cook, stirring, for 1 minute or until fragrant. Stir in your stock and honey until well combined.

2. Reduce the heat to low. Add your cabbage and cook, partially covered and stirring occasionally, for 15 minutes or until the cabbage is very tender.

3. Remove the pan from the heat and stir through your onion and apple. Season with sea salt and freshly ground black pepper. Transfer to a serving bowl. Serve.

SERVES: 6

50g butter
1 teaspoon cumin seeds
¼ cup chicken stock (homemade see recipe page 51 or store bought organic)
2 teaspoons honey
500g green cabbage, thinly sliced
2 green onions, thinly sliced
1 red apple, seeds removed and cut into matchsticks

   (VG)

Blistered Capsicum & Tomato

Time to prepare: 15 minutes
Time to cook: 13 minutes

1. Preheat your char-grill pan or barbecue char-grill plate over a high heat.
2. Place your oil, garlic, black pepper and rosemary into a large heatproof bowl, then stir until well combined. Season with sea salt.
3. Char-grill your capsicum, skin side facing down, for 5 minutes or until the skins are lightly charred. Turn over and char-grill for another 2 minutes or until the capsicum are just tender. Transfer your capsicum to the oil mixture in the bowl, then toss gently to combine. Set aside.
4. Char-grill your tomato, skin side facing down, for 1 minute or until the skins are lightly charred. Turn over and char-grill for another 1 minute or until just starting to soften. Transfer to the oil and capsicum mixture in bowl, then toss gently to combine. Season with sea salt. Transfer to a serving plate. Serve warm.

SERVES: 6

½ cup avocado oil
2 cloves garlic, peeled and thinly sliced
1 teaspoon ground black pepper
½ small bunch fresh rosemary, leaves picked
1 red capsicum, cut into 6 wedges and seeds removed
1 yellow capsicum, cut into 6 wedges and seeds removed
1 green capsicum, cut into 6 wedges and seeds removed
6 roma tomatoes, halved lengthwise

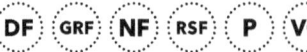

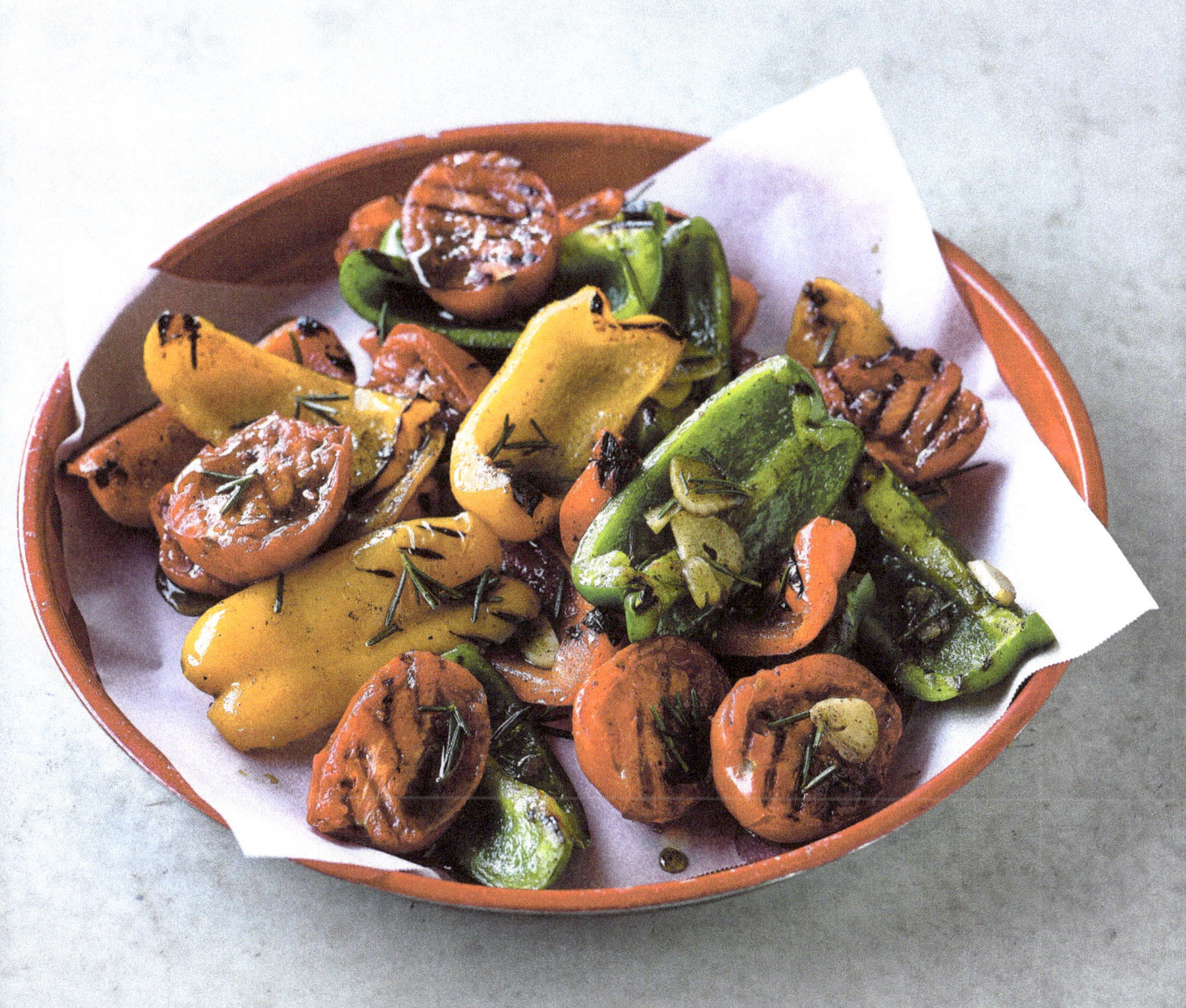

Index

B
Beef
Adobo Beef 99
Basic Char-grilled Steak 95
Beef Bourguignon 100
Gingered Beef 96
Meat-lovers Rib-eye 103

C
Char-grilling
Adobo Beef 99
Basic Char-grilled Steak 95
Beef Bourguignon 100
Gingered Beef 96
Meat-lovers Rib-eye 103
Chicken
Basic Roast Chicken 53
Basic Stir-fry Chicken 81
Buttery Chicken Curry 30
Jerk Chicken 57
Pistachio & Herb Stuffed Chicken 54
Spring Chicken, Stewp 44
Steam-roasted Chinese Chicken 58
Stir-fry Salad 89
Sweet & Sour Stir-fry 86
Vietnamese Wraps 82
Weeknight Roast Chicken 61
Chutney
Tomato & Peach Chutney 26
Curry
Buttery Chicken Curry 30

E
Eggs
Anytime Eggs 33
Fried Egg & Stir-fry 85

L
Lamb
Basic Slow-cooked Lamb 66
Lamb Salad 70
Lemony Greek Lamb 69
Make it a Slow-cooker Meal 74
Sumac Lamb 73

P
Pork
Asian Pork & Cabbage, Stewp 47

R
Roast
Basic Roast Chicken 53
Jerk Chicken 57
Pistachio & Herb Stuffed Chicken 54
Roast Pumpkin & Sage Brown Butter, Smash 133
Roasted Cauliflower & Pomegranate, Salad 108
Roast Pumpkin & Sage Brown Butter, Smash 133
Steam-roasted Chinese Chicken 58
Weeknight Roast Chicken 61

S

Salad
Baby Green Salad 115
Heirloom Tomato Salad 111
Lemony Greek Lamb 69
Lamb Salad 70
Roasted Cauliflower &
    Pomegranate 108
Spring Salad 112
Stir-fry Salad 89
Super-green Slaw 116
Winter Citrus & Thyme 119

Sauce
Basic Tomato Sauce 25
Lentil Pasta Sauce 29

Slow-cooked
Basic Slow-cooked Lamb 66
Lemony Greek Lamb 69
Lamb Salad 70
Make it a Slow-cooker Meal 74
Sumac Lamb 73

Smash
Artichoke & Celeriac 130
Carrot & Swede Colcannon 126
Roast Pumpkin & Sage Brown
    Butter 133
Smoky Summer Eggplant 129
Whipped Sweet Potato Chump 125
Zesty Avocado & Pea 134

Steak
Adobo Beef 99
Basic Char-grilled Steak 95
Beef Bourguignon 100
Gingered Beef 96
Meat-lovers Rib-eye 103

Stewp
Almost Meat-free 40
Asian Pork & Cabbage 47
Basic Stewp 39
Chorizo & Chilli 43
Spring Chicken 44

Stir-fry
Basic Stir-fry Chicken 81
Fried Egg & Stir-fry 85
Stir-fry Salad 89
Sweet & Sour Stir-fry 86
Vietnamese Wraps 82

T

Tomato
Basic Tomato Sauce 25
Blistered Capsicum & Tomato 150
Heirloom Tomato Salad 111
Tomato & Peach Chutney 26

V

Vegetable
Artichoke & Celeriac, Smash 130
Carrot & Swede Colcannon,
    Smash 126
Blistered Capsicum & Tomato 150
Braised Cabbage 149
Glazed Beets & Sprouts 146
Mushrooms with Crispy Chilli &
    Ginger 141
Raw Peas with Macadamia 145
Roasted Cauliflower & Pomegranate,
    Salad 108
Smoky Summer Eggplant, Smash 129
Whipped Sweet Potato Chump,
    Smash 125
Winter Bake 142
Zesty Avocado & Pea, Smash 134

About Tracey

I am a Sydney-based food publishing professional and a qualified Holistic Health Coach (IIN). I believe the foundation to great health begins in the kitchen, getting back to the basics – real food, trusted recipes and simple cookery skills.

The healthy recipes I create are tried and tested daily in my kitchen and are grounded in the two decades of food publishing experience I have.

My professional work features in world leading food magazines and cookbooks. A career which has spanned across the United Kingdom, the Middle East, Europe and North America.

My intention is to empower you with all the tools and tips required for recipe success, giving you the confidence you deserve in the kitchen so you too can truly learn to *love to cook* and in turn live a holistic, healthy life.

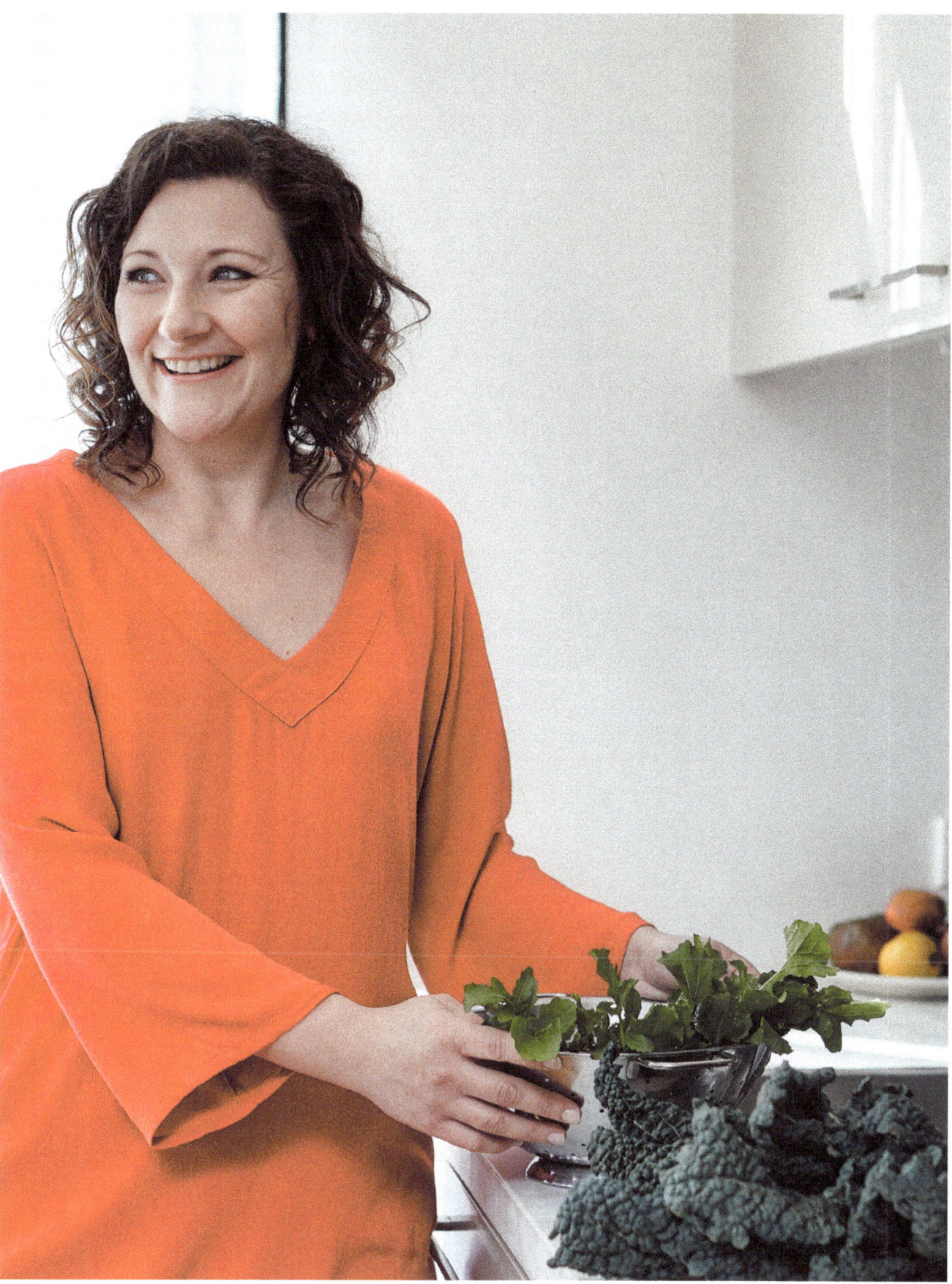

> *"I believe you can make Healthy Meals that taste great, are affordable and your children will love to eat."*
> **TRACEY PATTISON**

Love To Cook – *Healthy Meals*

Copyright © 2015 by Tracey Pattison

All rights reserved. No part of this publication may be reproduced, distributed, or transmitted in any form or by any means, including photocopying, recording, or other electronic or mechanical methods, without the prior written permission of the publisher or author, except in the case of brief quotations embodied in critical reviews and certain other noncommercial uses permitted by copyright law. For permission requests, email the author at welcome@getfoodfit.com

To contact the author visit www.getfoodfit.com

ISBN 978-0-646-94810-2

Cover and Internal Design by Hannah Janzen
Photography by Steve Brown
Food Preparation by Theressa Klein

Follow Tracey

tracey.pattison @getfoodfit
getfoodfit

www.ingramcontent.com/pod-product-compliance
Lightning Source LLC
Chambersburg PA
CBHW061820290426
44110CB00027B/2926